A Lump in the Road

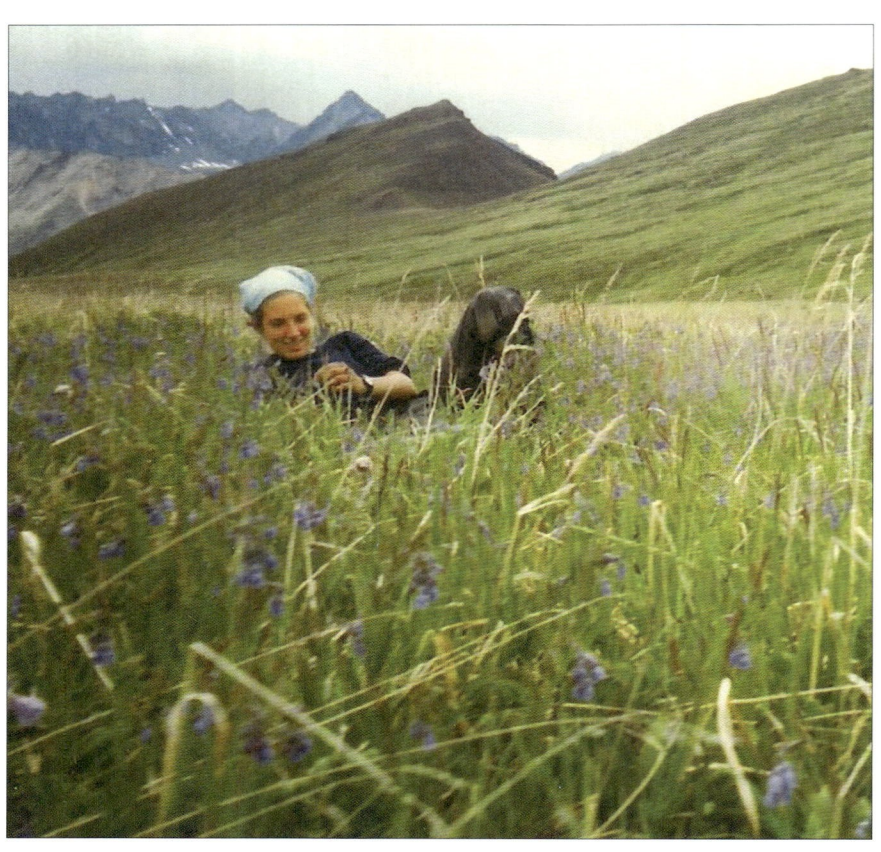

Sitting in a bluebell field in the Brooks Range of Alaska, July 16, 1996

A LUMP IN THE ROAD

My Personal Journey with a
Ductal Carcinoma In Situ (DCIS)
Diagnosis

By Kate Navarra

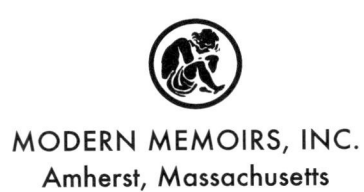

MODERN MEMOIRS, INC.
Amherst, Massachusetts

The thoughts, reflections, and opinions expressed in this book are those of the author, based upon her personal recollections and research. The author takes full and sole responsibility for all of the contents, including text and images, and regrets any aspect of the content that might be construed as injurious to a party mentioned, implied, or referred to.

Cover design by Moira Clingman.
Back cover image courtesy of Lake Washington School District, King County, Washington. All other images courtesy of the author.
Printed and bound in the U.S.

ISBN 978-1-09836-523-3
To purchase a copy of this book, please visit: **Store.Bookbaby.com**
To contact the author, please email: **alumpintheroad@yahoo.com**

MODERN MEMOIRS, INC.
495 West Street, Suite 1C
Amherst, Massachusetts 01002
413-253-2353
www.modernmemoirs.com

To anyone who has faced cancer, regardless of the stage,
as a patient, a friend, or a family member.
I see you and respect you.
You've got this.

CONTENTS

INTRODUCTION

May 2019

I thought I had things pretty well figured out. I was so many things. I was a nearly forty-year-old mother of two. I was a wife. I was a friend. I was a historian. I was an author. I was a stay-at-home mom who was rarely at home. I had a routine. I had a schedule for me and my kids. I could often be found wandering the various group fitness classes at the YMCA; planning classroom functions for my children's elementary school; or helping with a large or small project for the Parent Teacher Student Association (PTSA). (Who am I kidding? They are always large projects.)

Then I turned forty. As it is for most other people, my birthday was just another day on the calendar, another choice of restaurant and cake to celebrate the big four-oh. But just after I turned that ripe old age, I started a journey I'd never anticipated taking. This book is about the emotional journey I took after being diagnosed with Ductal Carcinoma In Situ (DCIS), a not-well-known, but fairly common cancer that affects over 50,000 women a year in the United States and has an almost 100% survival rate. While this latter statistic is good news, those of us who are diagnosed with DCIS live in limbo between being cancer survivors and not having had a "real" (invasive) cancer that requires radiation or chemotherapy and all the side effects. But the tests we endure are similar, and the waiting is identical, and the emotional ups and downs are heart-wrenching.

My diagnosis came unexpectedly, as cancer often does.

And while I, of course, never meant to have cancer, I also never meant to sit down and write a book about what happened after my diagnosis. My writing emerged organically when a friend, another Kate who lives across the country, asked me how I was dealing with being diagnosed with cancer. It was too much to text. And phone calls were difficult due to time zone differences and the fact that I found myself unable to speak out loud about all the emotions and fears I faced when I got my diagnosis. I also wasn't (at the time) ready to talk about cancer in front of my children.

Hearing my concerns, my friend said, "Why don't you write a blog?"

A blog? Like something on the internet that anyone could see? I thought about it for a couple of days and decided to start journaling instead. Then came the constant questions from more close friends who lived far away: How are you? Have you been keeping busy? Did you hear back from the doctor yet?

It wasn't that these questions were a bother, but it turned out that being able to report on my feelings, most recent test results, and my emotions in dealing with it all in a way that people could access on their own was a good idea. So, I put my journaling into a blog. A Lump in the Road was born.

Blogging quickly became a necessity in my daily life. I needed to be able to swear, to "say" out loud that I was afraid to die, and to disclose emotions I didn't feel comfortable sharing with my closest relatives and friends out of fear that they were as scared as I was. Writing—shared or unshared—has always helped me better understand who I am. During my cancer journey, it has been a crucial part of my healing process and my recovery.

As you read this book, please keep in mind that this is my

personal journey. Just as not every person chooses the same path on a journey, not everyone handles a diagnosis in the same way. In one year, I won a battle with cancer. I lost two boobs, but I walked away with a voice that was stronger than ever. It's that voice I share with you here.

Kate Navarra
Sammamish, Washington
August 2020

1

The Cliff

Summer 1996

There are challenging moments in life when you see a flash of what is important—the proverbial "life passes before your eyes" moments. It is then when you recognize what defines you, the instances that are so important they're etched into your brain. In times like this we often discover we are stronger than we ever knew we could be, but only after breaking into a million pieces, wallowing in fear and self-doubt, and finally finding peace. I have been to this type of precipice twice so far, grasping at air, struggling to hold on.

These precipice moments came at two completely different phases of my life with different expectations and different people surrounding and supporting me. The first was during a backpacking trip through Alaska at age seventeen. The second was during my journey with a cancer diagnosis at age forty. And while these two parts of my life may seem wildly unrelated, in retrospect they are quite similar. In both journeys, I found myself and discovered how strong I am.

I took a National Outdoor Leadership School (NOLS) trip to Alaska during high school. The decision to backpack in the Brooks Range of Alaska with sixteen other teenagers came quite lightly—in fact, I hardly thought about it at all. I signed up to go after a very difficult junior year. I suppose you could define me as one of those students who had a few good friends, but one who spent most of her time studying. (I honestly loved homework and the satisfaction of completing something well and on time.) But even though I thrived on academic challenge, in my junior year I took four Advanced Placement courses: AP English, AP Biology, AP Physics, and AP Calculus. The work never stopped. As soon as the bell rang, I was home making flash cards, reading textbooks, taking notes, and highlighting my workbooks. My mom knocked on my door every night at 6:15 p.m. for dinner, then I would go right back to studying until bedtime.

I felt compelled to keep up this pace because junior year of high school was a year of tests. I felt like I lost myself in the question of what college was right for me, the expectations of the people around me (family, teachers, friends), and preparation for the four AP tests. I was never any good at standardized tests. I could read, write, comprehend, and discuss just about anything in my classes, but when it came to answering a multiple-choice test question, I never felt confident I could get it right. There always seemed to be two correct answers or none at all. Studying for these tests did not leave much time for socializing or relaxing or finding hobbies.

When it came to decide on an activity for the summer after the SATs and AP tests, my mom literally held up three brochures in my doorway. I couldn't even tell you what two of the brochures were for. I only remember that I pointed to the one with the beautiful blue and purple skies with green meadows and white snowcapped mountains, not even reading what it was about.

I should have read more carefully, since NOLS would not offer the relaxing vacation I needed. NOLS is a nonprofit global wilderness school based in Lander, Wyoming that helps people step into leadership roles by experiencing the outdoors. It offers wilderness medicine courses and data-informed curricula so you can build hands-on outdoor skills through real-life scenarios. Participants learn the basics of packing a backpack, first aid, gear upkeep, and back-country cooking. Today, NOLS offers over 1,000 courses of varying lengths from two days to a semester in thirty different countries. The lessons in leadership are presented in the context of remote wilderness training on a thirty-day backpacking trek through untouched beauty. My first day with NOLS entailed seven miles of bushwhacking through the Alaskan wilderness, followed by a group meeting about setting goals and expectations.

That's some vacation.

My journal entries from the first day indicate more emotions than I thought I could have felt at seventeen. Overwhelmed. Hopeless. Inept. I wrote:

> June 21, 1996
> There is an unusual number of people who are experienced, really experienced. I thought I could handle these feelings, but then came the self-doubt and total fatigue. And this is only the second day. I guess I am just scared that I won't make it to the end.

Among my backpacking mates were young adults who had experimented with drugs, fallen in love, failed out of college, played drums in a band, tried to commit suicide, got straight A's, and were star soccer players. At first it felt like I had nothing in common with anyone I would be out in the middle of nowhere with. But in the coming weeks, and after sharing close quarters in small tents, I found we all had challenges to overcome.

Cleve was one of the NOLS instructors. He'd had an office job forever, he said, and decided he needed to change his perspective and liked what NOLS had to offer: being in nature and meeting new people. He taught us first aid and gave us leadership examples at every turn. Erica was another NOLS instructor. She graduated from Brown University and was not sure what she wanted to do in life, so she trained to be a wilderness and leadership instructor until she figured it out. She taught plant life and biology of tundra. Both Erica and Cleve were the first adult mentors I had ever met who swore freely and encouraged us to do so, as well. It was important to communicate respectfully throughout our expedition; how we did that, however, was our choice.

These instructors got paid $40 a day to lead seventeen young adults through untouched wilderness and make sure they made it out alive and well-trained to survive and be leaders. But they were doing what they loved. They got to see the whole group graduate from a course and gain life experience. They got to watch the transformation of young adults.

As for the other students on the trip, there were people who immediately stood out as leaders. Maybe it was because they were taller, or maybe they had an air of confidence. Eric, who was my age, was one of those people. He was a championship soccer player from New Hampshire. He seemed to have his life on track.

My initial thoughts about Brent were that he was quiet but strong. He was the first one to offer a hand when you fell in a river or slipped in the mud. And I did both of those things many times!

Jessie was a trained ballet dancer from Louisiana. Over the course of the trip, she sprained both of her ankles. We were constantly soaking our feet in glacially fed water together. At some point on the trip, she developed a 101-degree fever and "the mung," something our leaders referred to as a sickness including vomiting and diarrhea.

Casey was quiet and kept to himself most of the time. He was from San Diego and developed a great sense of how to cook in the wilderness. Casey was adept at making pancakes, cooking them over an open fire in one pan. He would make syrup using brown sugar and water. I remember once he attempted hash browns using leftover powdered potatoes and spices. He also got such a bad sunburn on his nose during the first days we were in the bush that he had white tape covering it in every photo we took.

Katie introduced herself as wanting to become more self-sufficient because she suffered from being stuck in a dependent relationship with a man who was not nice to her. She was so confident in knowing that she wanted to move forward. She wanted to be a massage therapist. She was not hesitant about sharing her feelings and letting her guard down. I admired her ability to share such personal things with a bunch of people she had just met.

It was like nature brought us all together. We were strangers from completely different parts of the country, with different backgrounds and experiences. And yet, in the breathtaking and terrifying greatness of Alaska, we were all the same in one particular way: we needed each other to get the most from the whole experience.

Each day in the field, a student was chosen to be leader. The leader's role was to choose a map reader and then decide the route. Everyone would have at least two chances at these roles throughout the month-long trip.

On my day as leader, I utterly failed.

My objective was to get the group over the pass we had stared at for three days and hike to the airstrip where our pilot would meet us with re-rations and fuel. The day started out wonderfully with a beautiful sunrise, a brisk morning, and breathtaking scenery. In front of us, we had a pretty easy hike along grassy hummocks and meandering sandbars. After walking a few miles, most of us had taken our outer layer off and were wearing just our long underwear with a fleece vest over the top. The sun peeked through grey clouds, promising a beautiful afternoon. We reached the pass and stopped for a snack. Then, I led the group down some rolling hills to the end of the Earth—or so it seemed.

There was a large ravine to the right that dropped sharply to a river, and this is where I discovered my fear of heights. Bad timing. After regaining my breath and stabilizing from dizziness, I suggested we could go back up to where we had come from and hike along a larger ridge over several drainages, rather than scale down the cliff. The others wanted to climb down the cliff and cross the river. Because I was the leader, I chose to nix the cliff descent (out of my fear) and climbed the rolling hills to look for another way to cross the ravine. My group's morale nosedived. The trail leaders decided to override my leadership (or lack thereof) and go back toward the cliff to climb down. What else could I do but agree? I was mortified and realized I had no idea what it meant to be a leader, which tried my emotional strength—failure guts me.

To my right was a two-story drop to gravel, followed by a sandbar and a rushing river. The river was clear and, in the places where the white-capped water broke, you could see clearly to the stony bottom. The drop to the ground below consisted of medium and large boulders, some as big as four feet in diameter.

Cleve took a deep breath and without looking at me said to Eric, "Go ahead and start down. Stay about five feet apart and make sure that you're never directly above the person in front of you. That way if a rock falls down, there is less of a chance it will hit the person below you."

Eric started zigzagging down the cliff. He was confident. He yelled back that he was far enough away for the next person to start down. Brent went next. After a few breathless moments, Casey started. Brent yelled, "ROCK!" and everyone froze. A boulder about a foot in diameter broke loose and launched down the cliff past Casey and stopped rolling right next to Eric's feet.

Those of us left at the top of the cliff could only watch. Cleve praised Brent's efforts to warn the others and told us that was exactly the right thing to do. They began climbing down again. One more friend started her journey down, followed by another. An instructor went next.

Then it was my turn. My chest felt tight. If I could breathe, I surely didn't want to. My right hand played with the toggle that hung off the bottom of my vest zipper. I needed to take one step. The first step is the hardest. That's how the saying goes, right? My hiking boot felt heavy as I picked it up and placed it about six inches in front of me, sloping downward toward the boulders. The one great thing about being in an outdoor leadership school with the people I was with is that no one pressured me to go faster. They offered encouragement and suggestions, but never pressure. In this case, however, I heard nothing. The sounds of the birds and the rushing water faded away. I am sure Erica, another leader, was praising my forward progress, but I heard nothing but my heartbeat.

Another step forward. This time I noticed how shaky my legs felt and how unsteady my knees were. One more step down. By then, I was far enough for Nick to follow from the top. We moved slowly (mostly because of me) and steadily down the side of the cliff and then I heard, "ROCK!" and looked up. There it was, a rock about the size of a bowling ball, skipping down the cliff toward me. There was a 50/50 chance of choosing the right direction to step out of its path. I stepped forward. It continued past me and made it all the way down to the sandbar below, missing everyone in its path. A few breaths later, I continued down, picking up my pace. The near miss made me feel oddly more comfortable after facing a challenge out of my control (the rock), making a decision, and moving forward. There were two more times that rocks came down from above before I made it to the sandbar myself, but my heightened senses and renewed confidence of one moment on the cliff gave me the strength to keep putting one foot in front of the other.

Finally, we had all climbed down the cliff, and it was the most nerve-racking thing I'd ever done. My left boot hit the sandbar first, followed by my wobbly right boot. It was more taxing mentally than physically getting down that cliff. Eric patted me on the shoulder and said I did a great job climbing down. But I sensed that everyone was still annoyed and maybe a little disappointed that we had wasted so much time with my indecision at the top of the cliff. Jessie strode up beside me and without a word, we walked together away from the cliff toward the river.

Though we'd all made it down safely, this was a failure like I'd never felt before. I had always been a high achiever— straight

A's on report cards, certificates of achievement in classes, extra-curricular activities and summer camps, and extra-credit work. I expected a certain level of success from myself. I was unprepared for the situation that I was handed, and I faced it without confidence and ended with a sense of failure. These feelings knocked around inside me for hours that day and into the next. It was hard not to be reminded of it when there was nowhere to go to escape the embarrassment of fear and failure.

Even if I tried to put it out of my head, the group wouldn't let me. At the debrief (which we did every day after traveling), it was made pretty clear that I did not act like a leader. One of our three leaders led a discussion about what went right during the hike and what could have gone better. It is gut wrenching to sit in a circle of peers and listen to how I could have, should have, would have done better if only I had, (1) taken less time to evaluate the options, (2) sought the input of the team, and (3) asserted myself. As hard as this experience was, it turned out to be a reality check and it provided life lessons that have stayed with me to this day. I came to realize that I had the wrong mindset.

I remember telling myself: *This is not a vacation, Kate. Far from it. This is a journey. And sometimes life gives you cliffs, not meandering sandbars. So, figuring out how to approach challenges like this is the goal—before you miss your chance to enjoy something.*

After three weeks of in wilderness training, we were sent off on our own, in teams of up to six, without instructors, for one week. "We will see you at our designated meeting spot by the Caribou River," our fearless and trusting instructors said.

Small groups were chosen for the last week of traveling through the Brooks Range of Alaska. My small group included Eric, Brent, Jessie, Katie, Casey, and me. Our task was to plan out our route, travel safely, and end up at the last meeting spot before we headed back to the road where the NOLS bus would pick us up. Instructors had copies of our itinerary and would know where we would be each night. If we failed to check in, they would know where to look. There was no way of communicating—no phones, no walkie-talkies. The wilderness training, first aid, and leadership training we learned the three previous weeks were all we needed to meet with the whole group. Each day would be a hike of seven to ten miles, depending on the type of terrain. We had to work as a group and communicate. We traversed glaciers and boulder fields and navigated miscommunications and differences in personalities. There were so many hours to talk, sing, chant, and listen to the nature surrounding us. We got very close with each other. At the end of each day, we came together after cleaning dishes to talk about highs and lows and to plan for the next day. There was always laughter, even after a tough day. We weren't just in the field with our comrades. We had each other's backs. We were a team. A family. It was not easy, but we survived.

For about a year after the trip, I kept in touch with Brent, Cleve, and Jessie. I am still in touch with Jessie. I even visited her for my first time in New Orleans a year after we returned from the bush to civilization. She and her family welcomed me into their home for a week's vacation. Every time we message each other, it's like no time is lost between us. I can still hear her voice, as we chatted and sang over so many hours together.

Twenty-four years later, I still remember the most peaceful moment of that final week. It was when we were walking over a pass. We stopped to sit in acres and acres of bluebells. It was a moment of complete contentment. The air was sweet. My hands fiddled with wisps of grass as we friends sat in a huge circle gazing at the bright purple and blue glacial mountains surrounding us.

A caribou jumped by us. That trip and that moment taught me to accept the now, to live for now. I sat in the sun surrounded by bluebells and friends, and I was not thinking about getting into college or test scores or what I needed to get done. I was just breathing the now. Walking down that pass was like walking out of something heavy. My steps were lighter, my heart more open.

At the end of the trip, I had one sprained ankle, two inflamed Achilles tendons, tendonitis, and trench foot. And strength. I hadn't understood what I signed up for, and while it took me a while to grasp that I was going to have to change my mindset about the trip, I eventually did just that. I found the strength to get through the physical and mental challenges of that first precipice and everything that we endured afterwards. The last thing I wrote in my journal from my trip was:

> I am the only one who has the power to change. Love
> the power from within. Be true to myself. Smile.

Looking back, backpacking through the Brooks Range in Alaska with a bunch of other teenagers was the first of two significant events in my life that have given me the strength and courage to be who I am today. The other one was cancer.

2

The First Step Is the Hardest

March 2019

The big "four-oh" comes with requirements—health requirements. My penchant for following the rules stuck with me well past my junior year of high school, so I did the thing we are all supposed to do—I made an appointment for a mammogram.

My doctor had urged me to do so when I was lying on the table, one arm up so she could give me a breast exam. "This is the year you start getting mammograms!" she said excitedly, yet sarcastically. We have a good rapport. We often chat about kids and getting enough time for ourselves. She is a doctor I trust because she is conservative in her testing and respectful when she listens. She hears me.

She warned me that there was a high probability I would be

called back due to an abnormality on my mammogram since this happens a lot when you are young and have dense breast tissue. Also, because this would be the first of many images made over the next thirty years or so, they would want a clear and high-resolution picture to compare with all future images.

The imaging office was in the hospital, a relatively new building overlooking a historic mining town. On the day of my mammogram, I walked into the first floor, where a piano played by itself in the atrium, seemingly to make patients more comfortable. People wandering the hallways were there for primary care, cancer treatment, pain clinics, rehabilitation, and testing. Others were visiting a loved one who just gave birth.

The imaging reception area was staffed by friendly people greeting patients with "Good morning," and "Last name?" I walked up to the reception and interrupted a conversation one woman was having about a new sweater she got as a gift for her birthday. After giving her my name, she told me to sit down and wait for a nurse to call me in for my mammogram. The waiting room was full of people of all genders and ages. MRIs, X-rays, and mammograms all waited for these people behind swinging doors.

"Kate?"

My heart skipped a beat, but I followed the exceedingly nice nurse wearing dark-blue scrubs to a quaint waiting room, which had a row of five changing rooms with curtains to the left and some soft, cushy chairs next to a coffee maker and TV on the right. It smelled like carpet cleaner. She asked if I had any belongings I wanted to put in a locker and showed me how to operate the combination lock. Then, she reached down into a warming drawer and picked out a top robe before leading me to a changing room.

"Change into this with the ties in front and we will call you back when we are ready. Should only be a few minutes. Any questions?" She was so polite, and it struck me that she probably had to say that string of sentences many times in one day. I wondered if I was the youngest of her patients for the day, having just turned forty.

After I locked up my purse and shirt, I checked out what kind of coffee they had to offer and sat down on the closest chair. There was a screen rotating on the TV advertising programs the hospital offered—bereavement services, outpatient resources, lactation assistance. It really seemed like they could have lightened up the mood of the room by putting on something like *Seinfeld* or *Friends* instead.

I looked around the waiting room. There was a woman maybe in her fifties browsing her phone. Behind me, a daughter escorted her frail mother to a dressing room, and I listened to her patiently assist her in getting her gown on. Her mother clearly did not want to be there. I projected myself far into the future, at fifty or seventy years old, back once again to get a mammogram to make sure that I was healthy. Would I sit and scroll through my phone? Would my daughter help me get changed in a dressing room?

The nurse came and got me and led me down two hallways to the mammogram imaging room. It was a small room with so much equipment in it that it seemed like it was a storage room. I sat on an oversized barstool chair with a back. It could be raised or lowered to position me at the right height for the test.

For me, the mammogram was easy. I have quite large breasts, and after breastfeeding both my kids, they were shall we say, saggy. Having them smooshed onto two plates, in two different directions, actually wasn't painful at all. The most uncomfortable part was having to hold my breath while they took the image. The team of nurses and technicians were lovely and explained everything step-by-step while making sure I was as comfortable as possible. The technician reminded me that many first-time mammogram-ers come back so they can get a crystal-clear image for comparison in later years, and that such a call to me shouldn't be of great concern.

I went back to the changing room after grabbing my things from the locker, put my gown in the bin, and left the hospital. I did not give the procedure another thought for the rest of the day.

As much as I was prepared for the subsequent call asking me to return for more images, I absolutely was *not* prepared for it. The woman on the other end of the phone had a calm voice. She did not—would not—give me details, but said I needed to come back for a different ultrasound because there was something unclear on my right breast. She scheduled me for an appointment two days later.

I drove to the same hospital, walked by the same piano playing by itself, entered the same waiting room, put my belongings in the same locker, and put on the same warm top robe—opening in the front. Another nice nurse technician escorted me to the room and performed the ultrasound, taking pictures as she went. As most technicians do, she avoided talking and held a completely blank stare at the screen, performing her duties while not letting me know if she'd found something terrifying or nothing at all.

She asked me to wait, and a radiologist came in.

The radiologist briskly walked in, opened up the images on her screen, and redid the ultrasound of an area on my right breast, just above the nipple. She pressed hard and moved it around, pressing harder. You could tell she was trying to get a better or different image. She put the wand down and scooted her chair back.

She just couldn't hide her concern. Her brows were straight, and her eyes were wide open, unblinking. She looked directly at me and said there were three spots in my right breast that looked suspicious and that they could either be just calcifications or something called DCIS. She explained that DCIS is Ductal Carcinoma In Situ, which refers to cancerous cells in the lining of the milk ducts which have not spread into the surrounding breast tissue. It is customary to remove DCIS cells to prevent them from becoming an invasive cancer that spreads outside of the milk ducts.

She scheduled a biopsy right then and there for just four days later.

Panic.

Fear.

What if...?

Four days felt like an eternity. It was like I was waiting to wait for more bad news.

Past a certain age, worry about your boobs seems like a universal experience in our society. I knew that many women who had been through ultrasounds and waiting for biopsy results would understand what I was feeling, so I texted a few close friends, two of whom were older and had been through this kind of worry and waiting before. Some friends offered to drive me to the biopsy or to just wait in the waiting room. It felt like I was being wrapped up in a warm hug when I heard these offers, but I declined, saying that it was no big deal. I could get through this. It was just an appointment. I think in the end, I didn't want company because I was so scared. I didn't want to spend the energy putting on a brave face for other people, even my husband.

On March 22, I went by myself to the biopsy. Little did I know that this was only the first time that these medical tests would interrupt the regular schedule I had with my kids. I would not be at school to pick up my daughter, and my husband had to pick up our son at preschool. It was my full intent not to let a change in our schedule scare them or cause them anxiety, so I just told them I needed to see a doctor. They did not ask any questions. I kept details to myself, probably more to ease my nerves since they did not know anything was going on.

There was one nurse and one technician present at the appointment. The nurse seemed to be there solely to distract me, and the radiologist performed the biopsy. Most of it was automated, which was pretty cool. They started the procedure by finding the suspected DCIS spot they were biopsying, which meant they had to squish my breast to hold it in place, take an image, then place the needle biopsy machine on my breast. They injected me with numbing medicine. Then they placed the needle core over the position on my breast where the spot was on the image. The radiologist pressed a button, and the needle took six quick samples for biopsies. Every time the needle left my skin, it left more numbing medicine in there (thank goodness!). They double-checked that the biopsy captured enough tissue, and the radiologist was not satisfied and wanted six more needle samples so they would have enough tissue to study. She double-checked that I wasn't feeling anything and did the procedure again.

During this process, the nurse charged with distracting me was regaling me with stories of her teenagers and how fast they grow up. I was engaged, but it was hard not to think of how scared I was becoming of missing out on things with my own kids. The "what ifs" creep in mighty fast when you are literally stuck in a boob-hold and know that once you walk away, you will just be waiting for news. I looked at her out of the corner of my eye and I said, "Thank you for distracting me." She winked.

After the procedure was finished, I was given two small ice packs (laughingly small, really) and instructions to put ice on my breast for the first day and to wear a bra for forty-eight hours so that my breast wouldn't move and cause the extremely tiny wound to open. I was also prohibited from any physical activity for two days and could not go swimming.

I walked to my car, pushed the button on the handle, yanked the door open, and sat. I was totally still. I held my breath. My hand reached out to push the car button on and I dialed my parents. And then I just cried. I cried fierce tears through sobbing breaths, screaming about how I knew they were going to find something, and then what? I pounded my steering wheel with both fists.

WHAT?!!!

How was I going to tell my kids?

I just knew there was something there or they wouldn't be doing all those tests!

There are only three people in my life whom I can honestly say I have lost it in front of: my parents and my husband. It's obvious why they're the lucky ones—they won't leave me. They will be standing next to me no matter what happens. They will be strong to my face and crumble with fear in their own way in their own time.

After about six minutes of totally losing reason, I said goodbye to my parents, blew my nose, turned my car on, and drove home. I took one Tylenol that night when the numbing drugs wore off, and for the next two days, I was never anything more than sore.

Even though I felt physically fine, I was mentally exhausted. During school drop-off and pickup the next day, everyone who knew what I was going through treated me with kid-gloves. "How are you?" "How are you holding up?" While kind, these questions were extremely overwhelming because the procedure itself was not a big deal, and I just wanted the whole thing to be over and done with. I just wanted to hear back already! I just wanted good news. I just wanted to move on.

Waiting was the hardest thing I have ever had to do. Harder than giving birth. Harder than saying goodbye to a loved one. Harder than facing that cliff in Alaska because it was all about facing the unknown. I think I waited five days total, with two of those days being a weekend where, of course, no one would call me with test results. Every single time my Fitbit buzzed on my wrist with a text message (which was usually some friend asking me if I had heard anything yet, or the school nurse calling me to tell me that my daughter bumped her head at school but was good enough to go back to class), my stomach would drop and all the air would leave my lungs.

I went through every emotional extreme. There were times when I caught myself holding my breath during the day. I had to pretend like nothing was wrong so my kids wouldn't worry, but I was completely on edge. It was a fear like I have never felt before. I had thoughts about lying on my deathbed, mustering the strength to write letters to my children. These letters would include my advice as they went through all the things I would miss in their lives: high school graduations, first loves, heartbreaks, successes in their careers, buying a house, having children of their own.

Maybe the deepest hurt in my mind and my heart came from

thinking of how much it would hurt them if I died from cancer.

The other extreme came to me in moments of mental strength. I knew I could kick cancer's ass, and that nothing on earth could keep me from living my life and reveling as I watched my kids travel in their own journeys. I would envision myself wearing head scarves proudly, knowing I was strong enough. I knew exactly the role model I wanted to be for my kids—the person they could look up to and say, "She beat it. She did it. She's my hero."

Extreme emotions made it hard to take each step—to walk to school to pick up my kids, to walk the grocery store aisle for food, to pump gas. Fear crept into my mind at the loudest and quietest moments of life.

I admit that I ate bags of chocolate (they put Easter candy in the grocery stores too early!) and pints of ice cream. It's OK, none of it stayed with me! I couldn't keep food in my body from all the anxiety and stress. Every time I ate, I would have to run to the bathroom.

Several months before, I had started dragging two friends, Andrea and Ashley, to "boot camp" at the local YMCA. It was an hour-long class with ten to twelve stations, two to three times around. It mostly worked on strength training, but some instructors add cardio or high-intensity stations. It was a great workout, made even more tolerable (and dare I say, fun!) with fun people. One class we took was a bit more relaxed, where we could goof off a bit and maybe dance instead of doing jumping jacks. The instructor was good with that because it still got the heart rate up. Plus, who could not smile while we danced? I really wish we had video—it would be like watching a rave dancer do jazzercise, but with gusto and flare and rhythm.

Andrea, Ashley, and I were always in a group at a station,

either by ourselves or with one other person. "Don't start at the running part! I hate running!" Andrea would say every time.

"Don't start at the rest station! That's lame!" I would say.

Ashley would have us start at the burpee or push-up station. Our discussions were always lively, and usually inappropriate. Once we talked about someone who was having surgery for testicular cancer. And while this is not at all funny, we gave him several inappropriate nicknames, which Ashley said he would enjoy. We often talked about how dramatic PTSA was, or how difficult it was to get one of our kids to do homework. We talked about vacations. We talked about work and how Ashley was going to save the world, one troubled kid at a time. We probably annoyed our fellow boot camp members with our constant gabbing. We probably seemed exclusive, but we weren't. It was a comfortably uncomfortable hour out of a week where we could just be.

We knew each other really well, and these friends were some of the people who ended up getting me through a rough time during my wait for my biopsy results. Andrea and Ashley were extra vigilant with distractions and humor. They are funny gals, but it was during each transition from one station to another where we would dance, skip, or run, sometimes making fun of each other. My Fitbit around my wrist was connected via Bluetooth to my phone, and while I didn't have my phone with me when I was working out in class, I was keenly aware of the people trying to reach me. I was still waiting. Every time it buzzed, I would whip my wrist around to see the screen. Was it a phone call? No, just a text with a friend asking, "Any news yet?"

Not super helpful. "Thank you for asking," I would say out loud, and neither friend would miss a beat and say, "Someone is checking in on you. That's so nice."

I would roll my eyes. Even though I agreed, it made my

stomach lurch each time my wrist vibrated. It was exhausting. Then I would get a phone call, drop my weights or ball, and dash to the water fountain with all my things to check my phone, thinking, *Who is it? Is it THE call?*

No. Not this time.

When?

Andrea got us matching headbands and wristbands ("These are to wipe away sweat from your brow" she said) so we could liven things up at the gym a bit. Then I bought us matching workout shirts that said, "I am stronger than you think." Because we are, and honestly, I needed the reminder.

I pushed myself harder than I ever have in my life in these classes while I was waiting for my biopsy results. Maybe out of fear. Maybe to see how strong I could be. Maybe because I've never needed to be stronger in my life. Maybe because I knew that if I needed to have surgery, I would probably be unable to exercise for an undetermined amount of time. Maybe it was because of all of that. One thing I can say for certain is that those classes and the time with my friends saved my sanity and made me look forward to something when I didn't have anything else to look forward to. I did it for myself. Because I didn't know what was going to happen next.

3

The Bump in the Road

March 27, 2019

After five days of waiting, I was just starting to forget that I was anticipating a phone call. I was standing at the playground after school with Andrea and Ashley and the kids. The kids were playing with sticks. We kept reminding them not to hit each other with them. They wandered around the playground and over to the trees beyond the parking lot.

My phone rang and it was my primary-care doctor. "Oh," I said, breathing out deeply, and I stepped away to answer the phone. The familiar sound of my doctor's voice filled my right ear. My heartbeat sped up.

She said, "Hey. I wanted to call you before anyone else did. I've been watching my computer for the email, and your test results came back. I wanted to call you so that you could cry and scream and then have time to breathe."

"OK," I said, holding my breath.

"They came back positive," my doctor continued. "You have DCIS. Good news is that you are going to be OK. Bad news is that the next couple of months are going to absolutely suck."

"OK," I said, exhaling. I took a few steps forward.

My doctor filled the silence, "I wanted you to hear it from me because I care about you, and I need you to know that you are going to be OK. And to remind you that even though you may not be seeing me, I will be watching all that goes on, and I am here. So, they are going to call you in a couple of hours, and they are going to give you a lot of information. Write it down. Then think about questions and call them back. And don't forget to breathe."

"Thank you for calling me yourself. I really appreciate it," I said. "I will be OK. I will be OK." Then I hung up. I didn't even say goodbye. By then I had walked to a bench and sat down. I remember glancing over at my friends, who were looking in my direction. I gave them a thumbs down, so that they knew it was the phone call I was (we all were) waiting for. I wasn't crying. At least I had an answer.

I took four steps back toward the playground.

I can't walk.

I can't breathe.

I can't see.

I collapsed to my knees.

There was silence.

Then, I felt three sets of hands on my back. I felt tears roll down my face. My hands were on the ground, feeling the cold, gravely concrete beneath them, and then forcing my body upright. I heard myself breathe again. I heard the soothing voices of what would become my village. My sisterhood. Another friend who happened to be walking to her car was the first to fully embrace me, followed by Andrea and Ashley.

They offered to take my kids so I could go home and process. I thanked them but said I was OK. In fact, in some ways it was the most OK I had been since the biopsy. I had an answer. Not a great one, but an answer. Something about knowing versus not knowing had a calming effect. And just like my doctor had said, I knew needed to keep breathing before the pathologist called with the next steps.

I also knew I had to move forward with my day for my kids' sake. My daughter had to get home to do homework before piano lessons. Life doesn't stop. Not for this. I would be OK. My doctor said so. Now I just needed to believe it.

As my day moved on and I waited for the pathologist's call, I found myself recognizing the fear I was experiencing. This felt like the cliff I faced in Alaska. I was facing a situation that I didn't want to be in, and all I could do was make choices and move forward, down the cliff. I didn't want to go over that cliff again. But this was cancer. I didn't have a choice.

The pathologist called. I had a pencil ready and took notes. She was kind and patient as she told me that next steps were: to have an MRI and possibly another biopsy, meet with a surgical team, and move forward from there. The MRI was a third level of checking to make sure there were no cancers anywhere that the previous tests couldn't see. The MRI would be done with a contrast that can see blood flow since cancer needs blood to thrive.

I FaceTimed one of my best friends, Lynn. It was so reassuring to see her. Her family has a long history with cancer, and she herself was always waiting for an eventual diagnosis of breast cancer since so many of her relatives die of cancer, though she didn't have a genetic marker. Her own health history is one of dozens of mammograms and biopsies, though until that point, no diagnosis had been made. But she always seemed to be waiting for it. She asked how I was. I answered honestly. I was overwhelmed but OK. I felt better now that I had an answer. I didn't have to think "what if" anymore because I had the IF. She told me she was going to check in a lot, and that I would eventually be annoyed with her. But she also didn't think it was the worst-case scenario. She wasn't too worried. She knew I would take care of it and move on. It was just a bump in the road.

I FaceTimed another one of my best friends, Meg, who had a lot of questions for me about the type of cancer I had and what the next steps were. Her mother had died of cancer a few years earlier, and honestly, I just didn't want to put her through cancer again. I tried hard to answer her questions bravely and clinically, though I did want to completely break down. She told me to call her anytime. We both have young kids, and frankly, knowing she would be there for me was such a huge relief.

The next day, the principal at my daughter's school saw me in the hallway and handed me a bracelet. She knew I was having tests done, and as we were working together on a huge project to get a new playground purchased and installed for the school, we had chatted about various procedures and appointments. It never bothered me that she knew what I was going through. In fact, as time went on, I found the support I needed through the friendships I made at my kids' school. The bracelet the principal gave me that day was a simple, with various strings of pink. She said now I was the member of a club of strong women. It was a wonderful gesture and tugged greatly at my heartstrings. It was a club no one wanted to join. But looking around me, realizing all the stories of women who were in my life daily, who have beaten cancer of various forms, it was a club where I would be welcomed and respected and understood.

Though it was no April Fools' Day joke, I walked in for an MRI on April 1. I'd decided I didn't need anyone with me, though several people had offered again. I was in the same waiting room for all imaging patients, checking my phone for Facebook updates and any PTSA emails that came through and needed my attention. I glanced up and saw a mom carrying a little girl, maybe five or six years old, who was half asleep on her shoulder. The mom was whispering to her that she would be OK, that they just had to take a few pictures of her heart. The child didn't appear to be well. I already lived a great forty years. This child barely lived six years, and she was having some pretty big health issues. And while I don't know the actual reason this child was there, it brought me back down to earth. I was jolted with perspective. I was healthy and would live. And while my kids have had their share of visits to doctors for myriad things, they were strong and healthy. I was lucky.

The MRI technician walked me through the procedure. I would lie face-down in the machine, with my breasts hanging down into clear plastic boxes and squished a bit so they would stay still for the eighteen-minute scan. Gravity pulled those saggers down so far, they had to move the table up. I think this was the third time in my life that I had an MRI, so it wasn't a big deal for me. I don't mind enclosed spaces.

"Also," she said, "try not to breathe deeply."

She asked me what type of music I wanted to listen to. I replied, "Does it matter? Can I even hear it?"

She gave me a blank stare.

I told her to put on whatever the millennials like these days.

Blank stare again.

The MRI lasted exactly eighteen minutes while I listened to (but couldn't clearly hear) "We Are Young" and several other songs by the band Fun. Afterwards, I asked who would call me with results, and she replied that whoever ordered the test would do so. By this point, I had at least three doctors who could have ordered the test. She couldn't guess which one did, and she did not offer to look it up for me. Before I left, she added, "If they forget to call, go ahead and give them a call in four days."

What?

Who forgets to call?

So, I waited some more.

What do we do when we are stressed out? Eat. The people who had been on the journey with me thus far, in person, via text message, and through video apps, had offered to help in so many ways it was overwhelming. I have never been a person who asks for help. Most close friends knew this, so instead of offering to help, they offered me brunch.

That I could do!

One day I had brunch with someone I met when my daughter was just six months old. Silvia and I had been good friends since. Though they are not in the same school (or town), our kids have grown up together. She is an easy person to be around. She is without judgment, and we are two very matter-of-fact kind of people. She listened to me outline all the next steps and possibilities. She asked questions. She shared her friend's experiences with a different and very aggressive form of breast cancer. We talked about how another friend was moving, and the progress her own family was making cleaning out their home, plans for renting it, and new housing options for a family move across the globe. We talked about other things because we knew there was a future to look toward. This was just a bump in the road.

The next week, I had brunch with two friends, Eirlys and Julie, whom I met through my work with a local historical society. It wasn't the easiest job, or the easiest group of people to work with. For a year, we had gathered data on an historic inventory of our city, researching and visiting all the extant houses and buildings built before 1942, which was the cutoff date for the county's designation of a "historical" building. It involved many hours of driving around, taking photos of properties, interviewing owners, researching, and entering information into a database. Let's just say you learn a lot about a person chitchatting while driving around (and making so many U-turns).

In retrospect, I feel that these two ladies came into my life at just the right time, providing me perspective, guidance, and a new way to look at life. At brunch, we talked about our work: one friend was still working on the inventory and the other was just starting a job on the parks commission for the city. I spoke about my efforts to raise money for a playground and my kids' elementary school. Both talked about their grandkids. Then we talked about my diagnosis and options. One friend had already survived an invasive form of breast cancer. She asked me who my surgeon was. She suggested support groups. She asked pointed questions about genetic testing. She asked about my thoughts on reconstruction and the steps to be taken after the cancer was removed. Most importantly, she and our other friend treated it as a bump in the road—something that once done, we could move on from and look at in the rearview mirror.

Of course, one cannot survive on brunch alone.

I met a friend named Melissa for dinner. We had known each other since my son and her daughter were one. We met in a parenting class, and we ended up at the same preschool. Melissa still likes to remind me of how I first told her I was going through all of this: "You mentioned it in passing at pickup when I was buckling my kid in her car seat that you were waiting to hear back from a cancer test. That's crazy!"

It was easy to be open and honest with Melissa. We had a lot in common. We both grew up only children and were quite close with our parents. We both had two kids. Our husbands both worked at a local software company. We talked about our families, where we come from, and how we met our spouses. We talked about other things, too, because this was just a bump in the road.

We talked about my diagnosis, made fun of boobs and all the trouble they cause. I prefaced one topic with the phrase, "You may think this is distasteful, but... I am thinking of having a contest." It was something I came up with in a moment of quiet while I waited for results to come back. I proposed that if I had to cut my boob off, I was going to get something out of it: I would have a game where my friends pay me $10 each to guess how much my boob weighed. The person who guessed closest to the actual weight of the boob would go to dinner with me, and I would donate everything I made to a breast cancer charity. Some of my friends thought it was great; others thought it was crass. Either way, it was how I felt I could do some good. Melissa, of course, did not think it was crass. (Eventually, she, her husband, and her mother-in-law entered guesses.)

While I was waiting for my MRI results, I felt a lump develop in my right breast where the biopsy was done. I was completely convinced that I had developed invasive breast cancer in one week. This is 100% not possible, and my brain understood that. But my emotions convinced my brain that I wasn't going to live to see my kids get through elementary school. Fear and the unknown are powerful things. After many friends told me to just call and demand (yes, demand) my MRI results and ask about this lump, I finally called and left a message with my treatment team. The team consisted of: a breast cancer surgeon who performed lumpectomies and mastectomies for cancer patients; an advanced registered nurse practitioner (ARNP) who would answer my questions about genetic testing, details of procedures, and other options; a nurse who could discuss general treatments; and a scheduler. I was in excellent hands.

A day later, after 4 p.m. on a Friday, the ARNP, Heidi, called me and explained my MRI results. I paced back and forth in my driveway as my kids played in the front yard, and Heidi answered a barrage of questions that had been looming in my mind. She told me that my MRI showed nothing in my left breast, which was great news and something positive to focus on. The MRI confirmed that the only questionable spots on my right breast were the three that the mammogram and ultrasound found, which was also good news. The bad news was that the area in question was about seven centimeters long, which is quite a bit of breast tissue to remove, so they were preparing me for the possibility of a mastectomy. Heidi explained that just taking the pieces out might not leave enough healthy breast tissue to look aesthetically pleasing.

Next on the list of to-dos was a meeting with my surgical team. Both my surgeon, Dr. L, and my ARNP, Heidi, sat with me and my husband for an hour-long meeting. It flew by. My husband and I had been working on a two-page list of questions, but we ended up being so overwhelmed by the amount of information presented that we could barely read off three questions from our paper.

The team was caring, forthcoming, and practical in how they addressed the diagnosis. They explained that with DCIS, you can overtreat it by removing the lump or the entire breast, even if there's a chance it will never spread, or you can undertreat it by waiting and watching it and possibly seeing it spread. There were no guarantees that DCIS would ever turn into an invasive cancer (one that spreads), and there were no predictors. I could live the rest of my life with the same amount of DCIS in my body, or it could turn into invasive cancer. There was no way of knowing.

My surgeon's priorities and mine lined up—we both intended to cure me of this. I thought of her as somewhat of a perfectionist, so, as my husband pointed out, we lined up well. Waiting to see did not seem like an option for me. I felt like I would wake up every morning and ask myself, "Is today the day my DCIS turned into invasive cancer, or am I still good?"

The doctors laid out the other options, and we decided to wait to do some genetic testing and another biopsy. I had been diagnosed with hormone-positive DCIS, which meant that the cancer cells had receptors for estrogen and/or progesterone. As I understood it, this type of cancer grew in me due to an abnormally large amount of estrogen in my body. I asked if I should get off my birth control pills, and the surgeon agreed it would be a good thing to do now and then revisit with a gynecologist later to see what kind of birth control could work for me. I also asked what caused this. The surgeon answered patiently that there is not a huge amount of knowledge about this kind of cancer because it is Stage 0, which means it is not guaranteed to grow outside of the milk ducts. She followed up saying that there is not a lot of research done because most women just take care of it. I listened and thought about all the rumors I had heard about what causes cancer: hormones in chicken meat, microwaving in plastic, eating too much soy. It was too late for me to protect myself from any such things, but I started worrying about my daughter.

I asked if it was genetic and learned that it is not, but the team told me that taking a genetic test could help decide future treatment options. If I tested positive for what are known as BRCA1 and BRCA2 markers, I would be more likely to develop breast cancer in my lifetime. (BRCA1 and BRCA2 are the genes that produce tumor suppressor proteins, meaning if they are mutated, the cells are likely to develop alterations that lead to cancer. Inherited mutations in these genes increase the risk of breast and ovarian cancers.) The test, which consisted of spitting a lot (I mean, *a lot*) in a tube, would be sent away to test twenty-nine markers for cancers of all different types. The most impor-tant ones for this part of my life were the BRCA1 and BRCA2 markers, which if I had them, meant there was an 84 to 87% chance of developing breast cancer in my lifetime.

Would taking a genetic test for the cancer genes cause more harm than good? What happened if I found out I was at a higher risk for getting pancreatic cancer? If the test came back posi-tive with the BRCA markers, I knew I'd make the decision that my boobs would go. But before we got to that step, however, we needed more information.

4

The Rocky Path

April–May 2019

There are a few situations I never even considered as possibilities for my life. Finding myself heading into a plastic surgeon's office was one.

I stood in the lobby for twenty minutes waiting for the slowest elevator on earth. When I finally reached the office, the waiting room was full of people who were there for anything from Botox for incontinence to eyebrow lifts and chin tucks. Something called CoolSculpting advertised in a brochure in a plastic holder on the table in front of me promised a decrease in my tummy size. I never thought I would be here, sitting in a room mostly full of people who felt the need to change their appearance. This wasn't who I was. I never cared much for appearances, and I felt that cancer was forcing me into doing something I was against for so many reasons. I just wanted practical, everyday boobs. Boobs that fit in regular-sized bras and bathing-suit tops. Boobs that didn't create a ledge on my front so that I could put a cup of coffee on them.

I was called back, and the nurse handed me a gown and told me to take my "clothes off from the waist up, please." I'd already lost count of the number of times I had heard that phrase throughout this journey. The nurse and a recorder kept themselves quite busy with a flurry of measuring certain distances from my nipples, and so many letters and numbers were chattered out loud. Next, a camera came out. "Don't worry, your face won't be in these, so you don't have to smile." I might have rolled my eyes. Um, OK, I wasn't going to smile anyway.

With a DCIS diagnosis, there are a plethora of options. This was the first time in the journey I would be faced with what I came to think of as a "tree trunk" of decision. I imagined myself standing at the base of a huge tree and looking up: branches and branches held more branches, each getting smaller until another branch would hold the leaves up. Each branch was an option. Each Y in the branch was a decision I needed to make.

If I choose a lumpectomy, Dr. N, this reconstruction surgeon, would rearrange breast tissue to give me a smaller breast and lift me up.

"Do you fix the other one to match it?" I asked, really having no idea what the answer was going to be.

"Of course!" came the reassuring reply.

If I chose a mastectomy, there was the option of having implants or using my own tissue to create a breast shape. If I chose implants, there were options for those too, like smooth versus textured, though she warned me that the textured silicone was recently discovered to cause a type of lymphoma that sometimes disappears when the implant is removed. If I chose to use my own tissue to shape a breast, she would refer me to another surgeon in her office because that type of surgery was not her specialty. Then she asked if she could see my tummy to determine if that tissue could be used. Huzzah! It could be used, but only for one breast. (I guess if I were fatter, they could get two breasts out of it.)

Just think! A free tummy tuck with a boob job. Lucky me. That must be my silver lining, I thought to myself.

I think the surgeon was sensing my unease. She kept asking me if I wanted to see "the binder of breasts."

No, no thank you, I did not.

It must have been written all over my face how uncomfortable I was with that idea because she finally asked if I was done with all the information I had heard for the day. I admitted, yes.

I was asked to stop and make sure all my insurance paperwork was set in the office on the way out. I met Tifni there, who was so helpful in taking care of the insurance contacts and answering all my questions about scheduling. I mentioned that I saw a local donut shop across the street and said, "Maybe a donut for lunch?"

She replied with, "Girl, you have cancer, you eat whatever you want."

I smiled and agreed. That was a first—someone had said I had cancer out loud. I don't think I had even said it out loud at that point.

We spoke about our kids and our plans for Mother's Day. She was hoping to go on a long hike with her daughter. I thought that sounded really wonderful—an escape. It was nice to chat about things other than cancer.

Upon reporting to my friends at school pickup that there was the opportunity to have my tummy fat used to remake a breast, they started lining up and identifying which body parts they would choose to donate to my cause. That way, there would always be a part of them with me, they joked.

By the time I went for my second biopsy, I was already done with it all. It was at the same location, same check-in procedure, same instructions for preparing for the procedure. Three people were in the room: a nurse, a technician, and the doctor. It was the same doctor who did the previous biopsy. We recognized each other. I told her that though I appreciated meeting her again, we should consider this the last time under these particular circumstances. She smiled and agreed.

The biopsy would be exactly the same, she explained, and then asked if I had any questions.

I said no, and that my recovery was pretty smooth except that I developed a large hematoma about a week after the procedure.

She said that was pretty normal, but that it was interesting that it developed so long from the initial procedure since usually there is a discoloration (which I didn't have) and then a hematoma just a few days after. She believed the hematoma developed so long after the procedure because I am a healthy and active person, but that it was nothing to worry about.

I told her briefly about the process I had been through and what decisions I was waiting to make based on test results.

She assured me that I had a great attitude about it all.

Didn't feel like it.

They put my right breast on the mammography table and squished it down. Lots of numbers and locations were called out, I was told not to breathe for a few seconds and then I could breathe again. They had to take a picture to make sure that the two suspicious cloudy spots were in the right position for the machine to take samples. The numbing medicine was injected. The doctor poked me to make sure I couldn't feel anything.

Nothing.

Good.

Two series of biopsies were done. Then extra tissue was taken to ensure a large enough sample could be examined. Then they put another titanium tag in to mark where a biopsy had occurred. I guess it was a different shape than the other one that was previously put there. While all this was happening, the nurse in charge of distracting me and I were talking about our husbands' favorite cakes.

You see, this biopsy was done on my husband's birthday— his 40th birthday to be precise. Life doesn't stop just because you have DCIS. One foot in front of the other. And I am lucky that he could take over kid drop-off duties in the morning so I could just get this taken care of.

Apparently, I was the first patient to not pass out on the biopsy team that week. While I had never been bothered by needles (I spent years getting allergy shots), I can see how some women would feel woozy after the lidocaine and the idea of a needle puncturing their breast multiple times. The technician referred to me as having a strong constitution. I felt really sorry that they had to deal with patients who couldn't tolerate such a test. It was part of their job, I knew, and with such a caring team, I knew they would handle those patients with respect and kindness.

I got dressed and walked out, then stopped at the grocery store for last-minute cake supplies. I was told I couldn't even go to yoga to visit my amigas there, as breathing deeply increases the flow of blood to the area, and that's what causes hematomas.

That was a disappointment. Yoga had started for me a few months prior as a favor to a friend, Julie. She wanted me to come with her to try her friend Sonia's yoga class. As a favor—because I always said "I don't do yoga"—I went. It turned out to be among the quietest moments I had had in years. My soul needed that stillness again. The moving meditation with breath-centered Viniyoga, located in a beautiful sanctuary home just down the street from my house, was permanently set for a recurring event on my calendar on Thursday mornings. It was a place that offered wellness programs, mini retreats to "rejuvenate body, soul and spirit." Once I got the green light to go to classes again, it became a safe place where I could share everything about this journey that I found myself on.

There were several weeks I had to skip class due to school breaks, various kid illnesses, and those previously mentioned brunch dates. The day I came back, I didn't hesitate to share what was going on with my soul sisters, as I think of them now. There was so much support and respect. They were already supporting my emotional healing when nothing had physically happened to my body yet in the course of treatments. It is so hard to explain the true lift my spirit got just by being in the presence of honest and supportive people.

Our instructor, Sonia, often gently spoke to us about breathing through pain or discomfort. She explained that by focusing on our breath, we could become more connected to (or less separate from) our surroundings. This helped me immensely in my daily life (I yelled less at my kids), but it also helped me through post-biopsy pain and avoiding too much pain medicine. I also hoped that positive thoughts would kick the cancer out of my body. I had been "breathing the boob," a phrase I used to direct oxygen to where I was hurting. I'm not sure there is any science behind it, but it was like I could concentrate and send positive thoughts to it through my breath. It was something I used when I was in pain after biopsies and surgeries, and meditation and movement helped me be more in the moment. Not just cherishing the time I have with my kids and friends and family, but really being there. As my seventeen-year-old self wrote in that journal, "Love the power from within."

It sounds wooey. And whether you've known me forever or have just met me for the first time, you'd know that wooey is not a description of who I am. But breathing and thinking positively certainly became a growing part of me. Once I was diagnosed with DCIS, I needed more than ever to be in the moment—for other people and for myself. Noticing my breathing and being more one with my surroundings helped with that. As my treatment progressed, I was going to need to breathe a lot.

Meanwhile, I sent emails, planned dinner, and did the other things in my stay-at-home-mom routine. I'm sure I picked up toys, as well. As I continued in my own life, I also watched people's lives evolve around me. It was hard for me to accept the excuses people had for not following through on things. They had a cold. Their spouse was working late.

I HAVE CANCER, AND I'M GETTING SHIT DONE!

That's what I wanted to yell... but I didn't. I just kept moving forward. But it amazed me how dug into our own lives we can get if something doesn't jolt us into awareness of another perspective. I remember a moment of intense clarity when I stared out the window and watched the wind blow a hundred-foot tree. It swayed three feet in one direction, whipping the branches behind it until they stopped. Then it swung back in the other direction, the green branches struggling to keep up. I wondered if it would snap.

I wondered if I would snap.

When this feeling arose in me, I would go back to what my friend Anna told me: "This is a great opportunity to stop and live in the moment." And I am really proud of myself for doing what she suggested. I had been in the moment so many times with my kids since my diagnosis. Sitting crisscross on the floor with my almost-five-year-old on my lap as we read a book again, and again, and again. This time, I was reading and thinking about the words, not just getting them out. We were changing the voices for different characters together. He directed the characters on the page. I listened to my daughter and felt like I was reliving my entire childhood in her laughter and tears—the joys and heart-breaks of friendship, the successes and failures of things like new adventures on the monkey bars, the joy in her ease of being, and the fear of not fitting in. Neither kid stops talking, ever, and I found myself about to listen to their chatter like it was the last time I would ever hear it. It wasn't, of course, but I hung on every word.

Six days after my second biopsy, I was still waiting for the results. I was also waiting for the genetic test results. My husband reminded me that no one ever called from the genetic testing lab to ask permission to charge us, as is the usual billing procedure, so I began to worry that the test never got there.

Do I call? I thought.

No.

Because while 95% of me wanted to know all the answers, 5% of me didn't want to have to deal with the answers and conse-quential actions needed to move forward. Waiting caused such anxiety. The quiet times were so quiet. Thank goodness there were so few.

But waiting allowed me to decide that I didn't think I wanted to have a foreign object in my body at all. Who was I trying to please? If I got rid of my boobs all together, I would feel guilty. About what? Not looking like a female ought to look? Practically, I didn't need them, but would my kids not understand why they were gone if I'm not actually sick with invasive cancer? Would they get made fun of because their mom looks different in the locker room when we change for swimming? Would I be OK with having every interaction they have like this be a teaching moment?

May 1, 2019

Results arrived via Heidi, my ARNP and contact on the surgical team. She told me that the genetic test results showed I did not have the markers for cancer, though there was a variance, which I was assured I should not worry about. She also shared that the second biopsy came back negative for DCIS. The tested areas were just calcifications surrounded by tissue that was altered due to hormones. In one biopsied spot near the already diagnosed DCIS area there were some atypical cells, however. Heidi told me I could have that area biopsied, though there was no guarantee that they would be able to know if the cells were anything other than "atypical," or I could have those cells taken out during a lumpectomy.

At this point, I had made the decision that a lumpectomy would be the best option for me. I wanted to be conservative in my treatment and have the least-invasive procedures possible. I wanted to look as "normal" as possible and start down the path so my journey could be over.

My appointment with the surgeon went well, as I got an overview of the entire surgical process. I learned that the surgery would be about an hour long. First, I would check in and be given numbing medicine so the radiologist could put bracket markers where the surgeon needed to cut, using the mammogram machine again. Then I would be prepped for surgery, given anesthesia, and wheeled into the operating room. The doctor told me I'd be home by lunch.

Pathology would take seven to ten days to come back. Given the amount of tissue they needed to take (quite a lot), I was at the limit in terms of receiving a lumpectomy and having much breast tissue left. If margins came back clear, meaning that enough cells were taken away surrounding the cancer, and pathology came back clean, I could go for reconstruction surgery, and two to three weeks later, start radiation. I asked Dr. L if I really needed reconstruction. She said, "It seems like if you have the chance to have perky teenage boobs, instead of forty-year-old boobs that I'm making a big divot in, you should take that opportunity."

However, if the pathology came back not clear, meaning the areas they take out didn't have a cushion of healthy cells, or if they found more cancer, then my only real option would be a mastectomy of the right breast. And there was still a 25% chance for pathology to come back positive with cancer.

I thought this was all over! I screamed to myself when I learned about these possibilities. I had thought I was over the scariest parts. Or at least the possibility they would find more cancer. This process was leaving scars for sure—in more ways than one.

After the appointment with Dr. L, I called the reconstruction surgeon, Dr. N, and got on the calendar. Another pre-op appointment with her, this one just days after my lumpectomy. It would take three hours to reconstruct my right breast and make the other breast match. The recovery for the reconstruction surgery sounded much worse than the lumpectomy, especially since I wouldn't be able to move my arms away from my sides for weeks.

How would I function? How would I pour coffee? How would I drive? How will I do the myriad of things I signed up for before cancer took daily movements away from me?

> I made the appointments and called my mom sobbing. I did not really care what my boobs looked like. I didn't want to have help because I couldn't lift a coffee cup to my lips in the morning. Cancer fucking sucks. I didn't want to do any of this. This was insane. Insane.
>
> —*Blog post, May 17, 2019*

My options were slim if I wanted to get through most of the surgery and have radiation started before my kids were at home for summer break. I felt like I had no other choice. People who have had radiation had been giving me the lowdown on it. It is no one's first choice in therapy, but it's necessary to keep cancer from returning. Radiation builds up in your system and while the first few weeks are OK, it's during the second half of treatment that patients feel exhausted. Some people have burned skin where the radiation therapy is on their body. Some don't. While I didn't look forward to it, I felt like this was the best plan for me.

Mom said she would fly up briefly for the first surgery and planned on coming back with my dad for the second. It seemed like a better plan to have more adults on hand when I wouldn't be able to use my arms.

The next day I took the long trip to Seattle to have my boob drawn on. The reconstruction surgeon was nice and quick and explained how she was artistically drawing on my breast so the other surgeon would use the same lines, which meant leaving fewer scars behind. One friend referred to the photo I showed her of my breast as a "battle plan." It's a pretty apt description of the lines and marks, drawn in three colors. The most important purple lines were covered in tape so they would stay longer (there were still five days until surgery). I was given a permanent marker to redraw lines after showering. That seemed like a lot of power to give me, considering I am not very artistic.

A few days later, I thought to myself, *I can do this. It is going to be OK.* I was still scared, but it was the first time in months that I breathed through my fear and thought about how I could face every setback with positivity.

And no, it would not always be positive. Some days, I had to throw Lunchables into my kids' backpacks and call it good. But one day again soon, I would be back to cutting sandwiches into shapes and writing notes and tucking them into lunch-boxes. Someday soon I would be back at the gym, pushing myself harder. But in the meantime, I had to do only what I could do to stay physically strong for the future.

Two days later, a coordinator called me to schedule a call where an intake nurse would ask me detailed pre-surgery questions and discuss surgery prep and anesthesia. Topics included what times I needed to fast, what soap to use, what prescription medications I was taking. While it seemed like just a few hours earlier my emotions were in check and I was feeling like I could do all of this, overwhelming feelings now hit me again. With the addition of another appointment—even one just on the phone—it felt like my plate was too full, its contents falling onto the floor.

It was time to take another step toward letting more people into my cancer village. I finally told my son's lead preschool teacher about my diagnosis. I could foresee some potential issues with behavior, maybe some fear coming through in his play. I hadn't kept people in the dark on purpose, but I was unconsciously conscious of whom I chose to drag with me on this journey and who got to see only the façade. I'd decided that until I had a plan and a schedule, I didn't want to let his teachers know. It wasn't that I didn't feel close to them—quite the contrary. We'd known those teachers since my daughter went to the same preschool, and they were more like family. But for a while I felt they didn't need to be on the emotional roller coaster, constantly wondering what the next test result was, or what the next step would be. They were with my son most days, and I wanted him to have a routine, uninterrupted by the drama that his mom was hiding so well from him. At this point as I anticipated surgery, I decided the teachers had to know because they were his pillars of support outside the nuclear family and our family friends. I was confident his teachers would be ready and able to handle him with care if he acted out due to sadness, fear, or just because of the inevitable changes that would come our way. I know that if he needed a bit of extra love, they would be right there. I trusted that and had faith in it.

Then there was the moment every mother dreads—I had to tell my *children*. They already knew I was going to have some sick parts of my breast taken out so I didn't get sicker. It finally happened one night a few days before my lumpectomy surgery. They didn't sit long after I explained more to them, and they didn't have any questions. But I had a feeling it wouldn't be our last conversation about it.

My daughter started having a rough time going to sleep. So many things were distracting her: she accidentally spilled Dad's tea; she couldn't get all the snots out of her nose to breathe right; she didn't have enough time to read on her own; there could be a fire alarm at school; Mom might leave her side; Mom might die.

She lay in bed across my lap and asked so many questions: "Don't show me, but what does it look like?"

"Does it hurt?"

"What is the name of what you have?"

"What is the next step?"

"What does radiation feel like?"

"Why will there be a sunburn? That's silly!"

"Will you die before Dad?"

And then she said, "I don't want you to ever leave my side because I would be so sad, I couldn't keep living."

I was absolutely gutted. But I had to answer the questions honestly, at her level.

Appropriately.

Without completely losing my shit.

I told her that I was doing the surgeries and intense light (radiation) treatments so that I could be with her as long as possible, to see all the fun things she is going to do, to see how she overcomes struggles and to celebrate all the little victories in life.

She wouldn't accept that.

I stroked her hair and said that I understood her feelings because I have a mom, too, and I know I would be so sad when she dies. I told her that it's OK to be sad when someone we love goes away, and that we have to remember the fun times we had together and the things we did. And the stories they told and the memories we made. I told her that those things would last until we die.

She barely accepted that.

At this point I had tears rolling down my face, but it was dark, so I hoped my daughter couldn't see that I was crying. I knew that if she saw me crying, she would worry more. I didn't want my daughter to worry about me. That was my job. She asked me if I was sad, and I said that I wasn't sad but sorry that she was feeling so many big emotions. I also told her it was normal, though, and I said I was feeling big emotions, too.

"We can feel them together," I told her. "And remember that if you feel them, there are also so many people in your life besides me who would open their arms and hug you." That was all I could offer her.

I held her until she slept.

Then I crumbled.

My scheduled phone appointment was right on time, 10:30 a.m. sharp. The phone rang. Amanda the nurse asked me what medicines I was taking, if I had heart health issues, and she gave me general instructions to fast for eight hours before my scheduled surgery. That's it. It was underwhelming. She asked if I had any questions, and then she told me to ask my surgeon the only questions I did have at my pre-op appointment next week, which were mainly about recovery and restrictions for the days and weeks after surgery.

The night before what I'd come to call "B-Day" (short for Boob Day) was filled with changing my sheets, picking out clean pajamas, and showering with soap that smelled like a hospital (this could be a new essential oil aroma that triggers anxiety). The admit nurse mentioned that it was unlikely I would sleep the night before surgery because of anxiety. I stayed up late to watch the *Game of Thrones* finale and ended up showering at 11 p.m. It would be a late night and an early morning.

I wrestled with writing my kids a note so they could wake up and remember why I wasn't there in the morning. Frankly, their lives center around my availability to them at all times, so my main concern was that they would feel completely out of whack in my absence. But every time I went to compose a letter, I felt tears well up in my eyes. Instead, I left a Post-it Note for each kid, reminding them that Grandma was in charge of getting them to school, and that I would see them definitely by dinner.

I woke up before my alarm. I showered again, holding back the urge to gag on the smell of that soap. I got dressed and stood in the hallway, impatiently but calmly waiting for my husband to make coffee. He needed to be caffeinated so he could make sure my nurses and surgeons answered all our questions. He asked if I was OK.

"Yes, I'm alright," I said. But I wasn't.

I texted Andrea and Jessica to make sure that they would not let my kids forget who I was if something happened to me. To remind my kids that I loved them fiercely. That's all that I could get out.

Checking in was easy. Everyone was so nice. We waited maybe eight (very long) minutes before I was called back for surgery prep. A nurse named Gladys gave me instructions and set up my IV. Since that was my maternal grandmother's name, I felt immediately at ease and wondered if this was some kind of message that everything was going to be alright. While I'm not a religious person, the spiritual side of me has developed a bit while on this journey, and I felt like I was looking for a bit of a positive message.

I was instructed to wipe down my entire body with sticky antiseptic wipes. Gladys took them out of some sort of warmer and handed me five packages of two wipes each. I took off all my clothes and placed them in a green plastic bag labeled with my information. This is where my personal belongings would live while in surgery. I felt vulnerable and exposed standing at the end of the bed opening warm wipes. The first two wipes were for my face and upper arms. Once wiped down, my skin tingled, and then I got cold. The smell was overwhelmingly sterile. I concentrated on wiping down my chest area. The next two wipes were for my torso and stomach. Then I moved on to my back, legs, and buttocks. It was the rawest I had felt in a while, physically. Once I was done, I could put the gown and socks on.

As I settled into the bed, the nurse hooked up an IV and heart monitor and attached leg cuffs that inflated and deflated to keep my blood flowing so I wouldn't develop clots. Next, they wheeled me back to imaging so my radiologist could put wire brackets around the tissue that needed to be removed. The same nurse who distracted me during my biopsies came to pick me up in a wheelchair and wheeled me to imaging, which was in the same room as both my needle biopsies and all my mammograms. Once again, the high-tech methods impressed me. While they had my breast squished, they were able to locate on the image the four spots that needed to come out. They inserted small catheter-type tubes with wires to surround the cancerous area. When my surgeon cut me open, she could then more accurately remove the bad spots and (hopefully) get clearer margins. I could tell by the discussions between the technician and radiologist that they were perfectionists. That helped put me at ease. Then, when the technician was wheeling me back to the surgery-prep room, I saw my surgeon and radiologist with their heads together, hunched over, looking at the image and discussing. The technician said that they had a great rapport, and I could tell. I had an amazing team.

I settled in for possibly thirty seconds before my surgeon came in to speak to me and said that she was all set and that I should expect the anesthesiologist, who arrived maybe two minutes later. After asking some basic questions about whether I'd ever had a bad reaction to anesthesia, she wheeled me away to the surgery room. Rather than counting backward, she wanted me to think about something positive and beautiful. She said that some people remember the things they dream about when they are under.

It wasn't hard to come up with a positive moment to think about. It was from Alaska on my NOLS trip, when we were climbing up the side of a glacier. There was the trust of the people who surrounded me and courage on my part. It was so clear that day, we could see for miles. The ice was so blue. (It ended up that I dreamed about making dark chocolate ice cream and sitting in the backyard watching my kids play in their treehouse. And I only remember this because I sent my friends a video explaining it in detail while still high on drugs after surgery.)

Once I got out of surgery and sobered up (only a bit), I asked for my phone and was immediately overwhelmed by the number of people who had sent me messages and videos to say they were thinking of me. Once home I was inundated with lasagna, chili, cake deliveries, flowers, cards, chocolate-covered pretzels, and bubbly wine. It gave me strength. It lifted me up.

I continued to receive many emails (some made me just downright cry) and text messages checking in on me in the days following my surgery. My kids' pediatrician had called to wish me good luck the day I had surgery. My dental office sent a card. My daughter's teacher sent me an email and good thoughts and let me know how my daughter was doing handling my surgery. Some other parents from school sent emails making sure I had everything I needed.

Over the next couple of days, people took my children to their house for playdates so I could rest. They dropped off more food. I was called a "machine" by those who had seen me, shocked that I was up and walking around. I would like to say that it's just my constitution, that I'm built strong, and I think that it had something to do with my fitness level. Three years earlier, I had lost forty pounds. After two kids, I needed to make a change. I was tired of being stuck looking like I did and feeling tired. I wanted to be around for my kids for as long as I could, see them graduate, see what careers they would choose, see if they would have a family. And I wanted to be fit enough to keep up with them— they are so active! They barely sit down unless they have a fever, and sometimes not even then. So, I got into Weight Watchers, which worked well for me because I am a Type-A tracker and thrive on the accountability and rules. And then I started turbo-kick and core-strengthening classes. It seemed easy as long as I stayed on plan.

But there is a part of my personality that doesn't allow me to rest. I've heard the suggestion for as long as I can remember, "Kate, just take a break." But I don't. It's hard for me to be still. In fact, my mom recently asked which chair was the most comfortable in the house, and I responded by telling her that I've never sat in one for more than fifteen minutes, so I wasn't sure. I am just not good at doing nothing or sitting still. I never have been.

And while I understood that I needed to take it easy for my short-term and long-term health, I still needed a reminder, almost every hour.

The morning after my surgery, I walked my daughter to school along with my mom and son. I didn't have the energy to talk to many people, but I made it to the front of school and back home. My son allowed me to accompany him and his grandma to preschool drop-off. We returned home and sat.

I tried to stay on top of the pain. It wasn't bad, but I didn't want it to get out of control. Though I was prescribed OxyContin, I took only Tylenol. I was bored. I couldn't do anything that used to take up my time, like going to the gym and doing housework. My mom brought me reading material, but when I read, I was still thinking about how many options I had for treatment, and how tired I was of the waiting. I was tired of facing decisions.

Just two days after surgery to cut the DCIS out of my right breast, I had a pre-op appointment with the reconstruction surgeon. We were late (of course) because we had to drive across the bridge into the city while battling traffic and horrible drivers. My husband and I sat, uncomfortably, in the lobby of the reception area where people get tummy tucks and earlobe lifts. (I had no idea this was a thing.) I filled in all the paperwork, answering "no" to most questions. No medications. No allergies. No glaucoma.

Once brought back, the RN who was in charge of walking us through the details of surgery began explaining all the worst-case scenarios. No food or drink ten hours before surgery. If we lived more than thirty minutes away, we would need to get a hotel room for the night after surgery—

STOP, wait, WHAT?

No. Wait, what?

No. Why?

Apparently, they didn't want the person accompanying me to drive me home only to have something go wrong and then have me be unable to come back in time to stop, say, bleeding. These scenarios seemed more restrictive (and frankly, scary) than the surgery to cut the CANCER out.

After adamantly telling her we would be fine going home and that if anything happened, we would go to our more local hospital—double-checking that the reconstruction surgeon was licensed there—we continued with the reconstruction surgery details. An epidural would be needed along with general anesthesia.

Wait, what? Why?

I'd never had an epidural and didn't want one. I was scared I wouldn't walk again if they missed and hit my spine. Again, it seemed more extreme than the local anesthesia I had to cut the CANCER out. The RN would have to check to see if for my particular surgery, I would need all that.

So, we moved on. I asked about timing for reconstruction, double-checking that reconstruction would happen BEFORE radiation. I could remember that fact but needed to be reminded of why. She said that once the skin and tissue is radiated, it is less likely to heal as well. This could lead to necrosis, or skin death. If I decided to have reconstruction after radiation, then I would be less likely to heal and tissue could die. And that tissue would need to be scraped off. My nipple could turn black and need to be cut off. It did not take me long to cringe and physically move back in my chair.

I can easily say that I was uncomfortable with this woman sitting in front of me. I stopped her several times and said that I was sitting on the fence about this surgery because it was not required for my long-term health. She agreed that it wasn't required, but that it is highly desirable for long-term happiness and for feeling good about my body.

I was uncomfortable with that statement. So boobs equal happiness? No, I was in the wrong place in my life. No. Nope. Nuh-uh. NO BOOB JOB.

My husband asked if the surgeon could speak with us for a few minutes. It was clear to me that he wasn't 100% on board either.

The surgeon stepped in and brought us back down to earth. Dr. N was reasonable and put our fears at ease a bit, explained things in a more congenial manner. Her plan for me was a lift of the right breast and a reduction and lift of the left breast—to make them match. The procedure would take local anesthesia, just like the lumpectomy, and would take three hours or less, "Depending on how particular I get with making the tissues match," she said as she smiled and leaned back, letting me know that it was not a complicated surgery, just a longer surgery based on her artistry.

I asked again (and again and again) about recovery. Since it seemed that I was recovering pretty well from the first surgery, I really wanted to hear that the second surgery would be easy as well. And while I didn't get any guarantee, Dr. N said that people tend to recover similarly based on other surgeries. With the reconstruction surgery, I would need to take it really easy with house chores, since those daily duties like reaching for dishes and putting laundry from the washer to the dryer are often the under-lying cause of fluid buildup, which is detrimental to recovering. But she guessed that I would be up and back to relatively normal routines in one week. It takes four weeks to heal completely. Radiation would start somewhere in between one to three weeks after surgery, depending on healing and clinic schedules.

I asked her to look at my right breast, as we were convinced it didn't look so altered from the cancer-removing surgery. She said that it was quite puffy (looked normal to me, not red...) and that based on where the fluid was, there would be a huge concave divot on the front/top of it. So essentially it would look like a ski jump on the front of it.

Yes, I can live with it, I thought. *It will be hard to find swimsuits, and bras might be a challenge.*

I asked about other women who have faced this decision and how many decided to go with reconstruction and how many walked away. The surgeon gave an interesting answer: not many women are given an option for reconstruction BEFORE radiation, because it's a fairly new option—with cancer surgeons and reconstruction surgeons working more closely together right at the time of diagnosis—and there wasn't a lot of data. The reconstruction surgeon often saw a lot of women years after radiation who were not given the chance for reconstruction before radiation and later wanted to feel better about their breast aesthetics. And those women then had to deal with higher risks of tissue death. She said it was her hope that by working with surgeons who take cancers out, they could create a new process where women were given all the options before incurring more risks in the process.

The surgeon reassured us that I did not have to have this surgery. She said it was optional. She looked at me and said it was my choice and that I should take my time deciding. She was respectful and thoughtful. I appreciated that.

It was an overwhelming amount of information, and I felt like I needed to decide sooner rather than later. But for now, at least at this moment, the decision was not to decide. Perhaps I would get a sign.

> I can't do that. I have to decide. Look, I want this whole Cancer Part Of My Life to be completely over. Done. Caput. I want to be done with radiation NOW. No, YESTERDAY. Not because I don't want to do it. I don't, but not because of that. I want it to be over so I can move on. So I can think about something not as bad. So I can move on to brighter things. The sooner I can move on with reconstruction, then radiation, then DONE.
>
> It came down to this: If I was going to do reconstruction, it was going to be NOW, not LATER. Because it seemed medically irresponsible to risk losing tissue with a reconstruction after radiation. But this was my analysis, and I am sure many other people, given a choice, would consider the risks. And I have already

second guessed that decision. And I have already been told that is the wrong decision. I have also been told that it's a great decision. I have also been told that it is MY decision and that I will be supported in whatever decision I make.

I will change my mind and re-change my mind at least a dozen times before surgery.

—*Blog post, May 24, 2019*

I have a neighbor who used to work in the field of cancer-treatment plans. She was not a doctor or a qualified nurse or anything like that. But she constantly told me that what I had was not cancer and I shouldn't need to treat it—not with a lumpectomy. Not with a mastectomy. Not with radiation. Nothing. She claimed there wasn't enough science that backed up DCIS turning into anything that will harm you.

She was hard to avoid at the mailbox. Our kids went to school together. I watched her kids when she needed me to because I was the neighborhood mom who never said no. While I was fine with hearing people's opinions, this one really stuck in my craw. She was so confident. It festered so much that one weekend, along with so many other things going on in life as it continued, I broke.

And I raged—not *at* her, but *because* of her and all the things. I was at home with my husband and kids, and I scared them. Am I proud of it? No. Am I sorry? No.

I raged because I was not getting the help I need at home. No one heard me ask for help.

I raged because I was tired of waiting to decide a decision that will need to be redecided again later. I was tired of being in limbo.

I raged because I was exhausted. My nipple hurt (that's normal, my surgeon said, as all the nerve cells start to grow back together).

My husband threatened to call 911 if I didn't calm down. How was that helpful? He told me I was scaring the kids. How is that helpful? Maybe if they were scared, they would better understand what I am going through? Why should I hide all of it? Why should I pretend like I'm stronger than I am? Why can't I just be human?

At that point, I seriously contemplated not having any more surgery. None. Just not do anything. Just live with the ski jump that is currently my right boob, and hope that I don't get any more DCIS, that what DCIS is left is not going to turn invasive.

Because if I did have any other surgery, who the hell was going to help me? I stood in the doorway last week and begged—cried—for help and no help came. Kids ran away and left me standing with too many things. Husband was on a conference call. I gave up.

What would it take for someone to help? Rage?

—Blog post, June 3, 2019

My post-op appointment with my cancer surgeon, Dr. L, was maybe a week later. I was unable to take my husband because my son got sick, and we don't leave him with anyone else when he is sick. I didn't really expect to hear anything new, and we already had appointments with radiologists.

I disrobed "from the waist up, cover opening in the front" so the surgeon could check on my incision healing. She inquired briefly how I was and checked my incision. Everything was healing nicely.

She sat down and faced me and said: "So I have some good news and some not so good news. The good news is that you have no invasive cancer."

Enter the universe.

"The not so good news is that the questionable cells that were not biopsied were entirely DCIS. So, the margins on three sides were not clear." (Clear margins mean that the margin of unaltered cells is more than two to three centimeters. Mine were one centimeter or less.)

I think I repeated, "This sucks," at least fourteen times while the surgeon gave me all the details. She would have to do a mastectomy because there was not enough tissue left to save the breast. I asked repeatedly if she was sure (of course she was sure, she's a professional and a damn good surgeon) because it sure looked like there was a lot of boob left. She said that essentially what I had on my chest was a water balloon. What appeared to be breast was actually fluid.

The upshot was there would be no need for radiation. The down shot was that I would lose my right breast.

So once again, I waited for a new plan. This was NOT how this was supposed to go.

On the way home, I screamed. I cried. I screamed again. I yelled at the universe that this was not where I was supposed to be. I thanked the universe that I was not going to die. I apologized to everyone out loud that I was wrecking their scheduled lives. I screamed some more. I sat in my car, and I cried.

I felt like I was standing on that cliff in Alaska again. I was afraid of the unknown. I was afraid my body could not do it. I was afraid that all I could do was make a decision about something that wasn't my choice. All I could do was summon up the courage to face something scary.

While I gave myself a few minutes to break apart, to fall down, to reach up and look around for answers, I knew that the next steps were right around the corner. I followed up to meet with my reconstruction surgeon. Most of the DCIS was gone, so there was no real rush, but I could not stop thinking about the myriad options still ahead of me.

5

Decisioning...

June 2019

I thought I had chosen what to do. I was going to have a lumpectomy, reconstruction, and radiation. Now that a mastectomy was on the table, though, more options for reconstruction were open to me. I was confident that I did not want implants. Not only did I cringe at the idea of having a foreign object in my body, I held a deep feeling that implants were for vain women who wanted to fulfill some ridiculous ideal. In my case, I was trying to just fix what cancer had done to me and replace something that was cut out.

I had an appointment with a reconstruction surgeon who would do a DIEP (Deep Inferior Epigastric Perforator artery) Flap Reconstruction, which meant taking healthy tissue and arteries and veins from the stomach area and transplanting them to the breast area. I can honestly say that I thought they would just suck out the fat and reverse-vacuum it into my breast skin.

I was really hoping to get my silver lining—a tummy tuck and perky new boobs.

That was really naïve.

It turns out that this procedure is an actual transplant in which veins and arteries would be found in my stomach tissue, mapped, taken out, and reattached to veins and arteries in my chest. The surgery takes eight to ten hours. I listened to the step-by-step description of the procedure.

First, they cut a triangle out of one half of your abdomen, below your bellybutton.

They move your bellybutton but keep it attached. (This is the moment when I threw up in my mouth a little.)

They detach the fat and some layers of abdominal tissue with veins and arteries attached.

They place it in your breast skin envelope and sew everything back up.

Then they wheel you into ICU for twelve hours to make sure a clot doesn't develop (less than a 10% chance).

If a clot does develop, there's only a 50% chance that the transplant can be saved.

If you don't develop a clot, you go to recovery and stay over another night, and depending on your progress, possibly another night after that.

Recovery includes being attached to drains, and while I would be allowed to be up and around, I wouldn't be back to normal "for months."

It was overwhelming.

My husband sat with me in this hour-and-a-half-long

meeting. We had so many questions I can't even remember them all.

> My main thought was: it is ten hours of surgery to create something that does not work. It's just a boob. It won't work to feed a baby. It isn't a heart that needs to beat. It's not a knee that needs to bend or hold weight. It's ten hours of surgery for something that would look a bit better in a shirt. And what if I try and my veins don't attach, right, and we have to start all over? What if I try and I don't make it being under anesthesia for ten hours? I have two young kids and it's just a boob.
>
> —*Blog post, June 8, 2019*

What I thought would be the obvious and easy choice—using my own tissue instead of having plastic parts in my body—was quickly turning into my last choice.

We asked more questions—actually, my husband was more on top of this than I was. He, as always, does better in the moment when faced with information and data. I, on the other hand, have an immediate emotional response and then obsess over the "what ifs." I think my brain turned off when the surgeon talked about moving my bellybutton and then putting it back in place. By now I was so grossed out by relocating bellybuttons, losing nipples, and drains, that I couldn't fathom anything but throwing my hands up, screaming, and walking out.

Since the details of the meeting were garbled up with raw emotion, the most I got out of the information was that there were several stages in front of me, and that meant I had the most options. I could still change my mind.

First, mastectomy. This involved general anesthesia, an overnight stay, and a drain.

One to three weeks later, I could do an outpatient procedure to insert an expander into my right breast where the

DCIS-affected tissue had been removed, which sits in place to keep the skin from retracting. Every few weeks the expander is filled with a bit more with saline so it expands to the preferred size.

If I chose, I could have the left breast lifted and reduced at the same time the expander was inserted.

Three to four months later, they could either put in an implant or do the tissue transplant.

My options were still all open. I could even test drive the expander, and if it didn't bother me, it's likely that an implant wouldn't either. Apparently, an implant is more comfortable than an expander.

The schedule coordinator in the office handed me a sheet of paper with a date and time of a support group. It would be somewhere I could meet people who had made these different decisions and could feel free to ask what it was really like. I guessed that was where I would go next.

I cried on the way home. My husband drove us back over the bridge, and I just cried. After a few deep breaths, I said, "I need you to be honest. If you had to choose for you, what would you do?" Though I knew and understood that it was my—and only my—decision, I needed to get out of my own head. I needed to hear the opinion of someone else who had all the information I had been given. And though he isn't a woman and does not have cancer, he had to have an opinion.

He looked at me out of the corner of his eye and said, "Really?"

I nodded.

He told me that he would have the implants.

I think I gasped because I just didn't think that would be his answer.

He then asked me, "How different are implants than a tooth

filling? Or contact lenses? A pacemaker?"

Also, he pointed out, implants are reversible, so in that sense they are less invasive.

It was definitely a shock to hear.

> As I felt swallowed up by information, I found that I hated myself for going through this. I was drowning. I couldn't breathe. The water is so far over my head I can barely see shimmers of light. These feelings bubble up, often out of nowhere. In moments of quiet. In moments of noise. In just moments.
>
> I hated myself and I didn't ever want to roll out of bed in the morning. Each morning, I opened my eyes and felt a wave of dread. I hadn't made up my mind. I didn't like any of the options. I wouldn't be happy with anything I chose. If I ever chose.
>
> —*Blog post, June 8, 2019*

The first option I tried to weigh was a mastectomy with no reconstruction. I would have one size DDDD breast and one flat side. A solution for dealing with this choice in day-to-day life would be to wear a prosthetic that fit into a bra or swimsuit. It would be a constant reminder that I have no breast. Would it be hard to wear a bra? Run? Swim? Shower? As much as I rejected impossible ideals about beauty, I knew that looks are an important part of feeling good about yourself, and feeling good about yourself is important to being happy and confident.

> The second option was a mastectomy and an implant. A boob job? Just to look better? It's not like my health requires a boob. I don't need them anymore to feed babies. It's something foreign in my body. Some cause lymphoma. It may move when I work out. It's a foreign object in my body. But is it different than a tooth filling? Or a pacemaker? It isn't needed to save my life.
>
> —*Blog post, June 8, 2019*

A third option was a mastectomy and DIEP Flap Surgery. It might not work, and then I'd have to start all over. It would be two places that I would be cut open. I might not heal well in my tummy. (I heard any type of abdominal surgery has lasting effects.) But it wouldn't be a foreign object. It would, however, be ten hours of surgery for something that won't ever do anything special.

I felt frozen. Stuck. I just wanted to be done so I could move on. The process was taking a toll. I felt like any decision I could make was not the one for me. Furthermore, it was like having so many choices about my treatment halted me in every aspect of my life. I had trouble figuring out what to make for dinner, if we should go swimming on the weekends, if we should have a movie night. It suddenly felt like none of these options were ones I wouldn't regret.

At the same time, I knew that I was not going to have to fight for my life. I was lucky with the diagnosis of noninvasive cancer. I wouldn't have to face radiation. I wouldn't have to go through chemotherapy. I just had these decisions to face. While they were not life or death, I wanted to make a decision one time to make sure I had the best quality of life for the future.

I summoned the courage to ask people about their boobs. One woman who I attended yoga with and who was a breast cancer survivor had mentioned that it was just a bump in the road, no big deal, that "This too shall pass," as she jiggled her boobs and said, "These are fake."

I finally asked her if I could ask her more about her boobs. She obliged graciously and honestly. Her boobs were implants. Saline. She was on her second set—the first one lasted thirteen years, and she said she was rough on them, meaning that she didn't treat her implants gingerly. She did all her normal activities—yoga, exercise, and so on—and they behaved like "normal breasts." She explained that one day in the shower she noticed that one breast was deflated, and so she had to get that one fixed.

"No big deal," she said.

It was an outpatient procedure to fix, and she described it as a kind of unzipping of her skin and replacing the implant and zipping it back up. She spoke of it more as a procedure and not as a traumatic event. She had a great attitude.

She also mentioned that she waited a year (with a lot of flappy, loose skin on her chest) after having her double mastectomy, and she tried the prosthesis and wasn't happy. While it was years ago, she couldn't find any prosthetic that was comfortable. She said her flappy skin showed in everything she wore. Nothing she put on looked right and she didn't feel good about herself. And while I was sure there had been many improvements to undergarments and outer garments in twenty years, I thought this was something to consider, especially since I only had one side to deal with.

> It was in this safe space that I first said out loud, "I am done with having big boobs. Why can't I have smaller ones I've always wanted." I was afraid to say it until then. Maybe I was afraid to feel that if I am being made to go through this, why can't I have a choice. Why can't I have something I want. I'm not sure I knew I wanted this but if I had to have it, maybe I get to choose smaller boobs that I don't have to deal with. Honestly, I've been wearing compression bras (sports bras, if you will) since fifth grade. I've had the voluptuous boobs. I can be done with them.
>
> —*Blog post, June 19, 2019*

I made it to a support group in Seattle, hosted by the reconstruction surgeon's office. It was led by a nurse who works with the reconstruction doctors and a therapist who supports cancer patients. There were ten women in the room. We went around the circle and introduced ourselves and shared our experience. Of those women, not one had the same journey. There was a woman who was diagnosed with Stage 1 breast cancer in 2005 and decided on a double mastectomy, chemo, radiation, and a DIEP Flap Surgery. There was a woman diagnosed with invasive ductal carcinoma and had a double mastectomy and radiation. She had not yet decided on a reconstruction option but was DONE with her prosthetics. There was a woman with benign tumors that just kept growing back who eventually decided on a mastectomy and then reconstruction with silicone implants. There was a woman who had a mastectomy on her left breast and had been adjusting her clothing for over a year and was so tired of it and decided to do a DIEP Flap Surgery as well. There was a woman who had a lateral flap tissue transplant and an implant, meaning that she used her back tissue to create a breast skin envelope that was strong enough to support an implant because the skin on her breast had undergone radiation.

There was so much strength and courage and honesty in the room. It was an open, respectful, honest space to share concerns about dealing with our diagnoses.

There was also show-and-tell. And with all due respect for the courage it took for those women to open their shirts to anyone who walked into that meeting, those breasts looked just lovely.

The following morning, I had what I determined ahead of time would be my last consultation meeting with Dr. N. She welcomed me back, though I felt like I was boomeranging all over that reconstruction office. I told her I couldn't do the DIEP Flap

Surgery. I admitted it was just too much. She said she understood my decision and reiterated that nothing we did now had to be a Forever Decision. Everything we did could be undone. An implant could always be taken out. I could always try a DIEP Flap Surgery in the future.

I asked her if we could do just one surgery—the mastectomy and implant directly. She said in my case, it was an option because I had large breasts and healthy breast skin. If I put in implants that were smaller than my breast was now, it would not be a problem. I chose saline implants. She said those would offer a slightly less firm, slightly more natural line, which, given my age, and the fact that I had breastfed my babies, would make sense for aesthetics.

She asked what size I wanted to be. I gave her a blank stare, and she smiled. I couldn't have been the only person who didn't know the answer to this question. I told her that I wanted breasts that would fit my body shape, but that would be smaller than the ones I had. She measured the width of my chest across from each armpit and looked at the natural curve of my body. She said that 280–300 ccs would fit the natural shape of my body. I said that sounded fine, not really knowing what that meant and trying to muster up some confidence.

And so, the plan as I left the office that day was to do a mastectomy with direct-to-implant and to reduce my left breast at the same time. The surgery would take, in total, about six hours.

It was the first time in a long time I took a deep breath. I hadn't felt this relieved in a long time. I left the office feeling like I got everything I wanted.

Well, not the cancer thing.

Cancer had to go.

And though I left feeling like a decision that I could live with was made, and that I could move forward, I also had the slight feeling that another shoe was going to drop.

I ran out of gas, literally and figuratively, as I was driving to my last pre-op appointment before my surgery, which was now scheduled for the 25th of July. It took almost an hour and a half to get there in a freak summer rainstorm through regular Seattle traffic. I was annoyed I was late, and I was annoyed I still had to deal with cancer.

> But I was emotionally out of gas. I was tired of waiting. I was tired of appointments. I understand in theory that I should not want to have surgery because of the cancer part, but I should be excited that I am having a lift and a reduction, right?
> I was not excited.
> —Blog post, July 10, 2019

I turned the music up. My playlist was ever evolving, and lately it had morphed into something that kept me going. Music had always been a huge part of my life. It's inspired me. It's challenged my thinking. It's shown me different perspectives. It's introduced me to new ideas. In the aftermath of my diagnosis, it was always at very high volume. The themes in music often helped me refocus my negative energy. Sometimes words moved me to tears then lifted me up. One song in particular had me in tears at the same time as it filled me with hope. This song was, "You Will Be Found" from the musical *Dear Evan Hansen*. It is a story of a young man who feels like no one is there for him. That was not the part I took to heart, though. Instead, I was moved by the part where he belts out that when he doesn't feel strong enough to stand, he can reach out his hand and someone will help him home.

This song spoke volumes to me because the universe had

given me a challenge: how to live with grace and not only accept help, but ask for it. This had always been something I failed at more than I succeeded, but now I didn't have a choice. There would be times during my journey when I would be literally physically on the ground, reaching up for help, and there would be times when I would do the same emotionally and mentally.

I was so thankful for my village of friends, near and far, who carried me home. Even people far from my zip code helped tremendously along the way. It was a huge comfort just knowing that my friends Meg, Kate, and Lynn could be on the other side of the phone via text message, FaceTime, or chatting, always ready to lend an ear, offer new perspectives, distract me, and tell me stories about their own lives, no matter what time of day. These friends from three different parts of my life, who I know are soulmates, were the ones who I could scream to, cry to, and sing at the top of my lungs with. It was these friends I gained strength from as I turned the music up.

I would need all the strength I could muster when I went into my pre-op appointment. Once there, I heard about the possibility of having a drain, the potential for infection, and the direct and adamant instruction to not lift my arms for two weeks. I had to let this sink in. I was ready to get this in my rearview mirror. I was ready to start the last leg of this journey. I had only two questions:

What bra should I bring to leave the hospital in? (Answer: they would provide me with one.)

Would they test the tissue taken out of the left "healthy" breast while they are reducing it? (Answer: of course.)

I signed my paperwork, I initialed dozens of pages of risks associated with surgery. I met briefly with Dr. N, who measured and re-measured me again and said about 200 ccs would be a nice size for me, though she ordered several implant options and would decide during surgery which looked better. A C cup. I had never in my life had a cup size of C.

This I should be excited for.

I wasn't looking forward to recovery. I didn't feel like I had the in-house support to help with the kids and make sure that their lives were kept relatively normal while I recovered. When I asked how my husband was going to help, he said he would be at the hospital and would take off work as long as I needed him to. He said there was no question about that. But it was the KIND of help that I was really asking about. I wanted to know the specific plans he had to make sure that the kids were occupied so I could nap if I needed, or where he would be willing to take them so I could get much-needed rest, whether or not I slept. His first plan was to take them on a family vacation.

First off—a "family vacation." Without me. That more than hurt. I thought doing something "regular" without me was thoughtless, and I told him so. Then, I was upset that he didn't understand I was feeling left out. I had cancer, and it wasn't making me feel better that he wanted to go on a family vacation without me. Wasn't I part of the family? I pictured a future in which I was dead from cancer and they were on a vacation without me. I understood then, and I understand now, that these were unfair thoughts, but my feelings and fear about the future were real.

Second off, I was convinced that what we normally do—travel across the country for two weeks—would be too hard for him to do alone. He had never taken both kids on a plane by himself. He had never stayed with both kids in a hotel by himself. He never had to help both of them do anything at the same time. I was ALWAYS around. After mentioning these things, he got offended that I thought he couldn't do it. I tried to explain that it was not that I thought he couldn't take care of the kids, but I was skeptical that everyone would be happy and calm.

He put off making plans for a while. In hindsight, I feel his lack of wanting to plan a vacation was likely procrastination and maybe not wanting me to have to go through the surgeries at all. He is not the type of person to overly think about or act on emotions, but as a spouse and partner I am positive he was worried and maybe even a bit scared, though he never let on in any way. Maybe his inability to plan was his brain not wanting to address the fears he had.

Honestly, I was so busy the day before surgery that I could hardly think of the details. In the five days before surgery, I had seen all the people who wanted to see me. I obliged, but mostly without desire to talk about it. I understood everyone wanted to remind me that they would be thinking of me and that I have help in place where I needed it. They cared. But I was done with it all.

> Last phone calls with doctor's offices and admitting offices upset me more than calmed nerves. They reminded me that there's was still a chance that after all this, they would find invasive cancer. The samples sent to the lab can still come back with positive results for cancers that they never saw on any scan. Honestly that makes me mad. Furious in fact. Why the hell have scans, MRIs, all that science— if it doesn't tell you anything? Why not just send samples of all your body parts to have them tested? Can you imagine sending tissue from your toes in to see if they have cancer?! I was so tired of waiting. And now I got to look forward to anticipating waiting until I actually had surgery. And then after surgery, as well.
>
> After all those phone calls, I opened a bottle of wine.

It's not the usual way I took the edge off, but I did it anyway.

—*Blog post, July 24, 2019*

I went to my last gym class before I would be on restricted activity for six weeks or more. It was boot camp, but not the class I wanted. It wasn't the challenge I needed. I cried in the moments of pause. I cried because I would miss it. I cried because it wasn't fair. I cried because, yes, I wanted to be able to do more pushups. I cried because I hadn't cried that much through all of this. I guess it was just time. I pushed through the crunches and the tears.

My parents arrived the night before surgery with a car full of food, projects for the kids and the house, and their own pillows. I expected them to stay for a while. I am an only child, so I knew they would stay until they felt comfortable that I could do things myself. I had to write down that I would allow help and that I would be a gracious patient. Otherwise, I wouldn't stick to it.

The quiet hours arrived before my surgery, the hours where I could not eat or drink and when the thoughts started streaming into my brain. The hours when fears of not waking up after a six-hour surgery set in. There were other fears, too: the fear of something completely unexpected happening, the thought of pending test results, the thought of being unable to get in and out of a car without help. Then there were also the positive thoughts of putting this all behind me and enjoying seeing it disappear in my rearview mirror. The thoughts of speeding up so that view gets smaller and smaller. And there were also thoughts that weren't my own, as I received the last few messages flickering across my phone screen with friends checking in and letting me know they were thinking about me just before I went to the hospital.

6

Bye-Bye, Boobs

July 25, 2019

We checked into the surgery wing at 9 a.m. for a 10 a.m. surgery. A friend's mom who worked at the hospital had graciously and generously arranged to meet me at the reception desk. We exchanged pleasantries, and she put me at ease tremendously. We walked only a few feet and then they called me back and Nurse Andrea started whizzing around taking care of things—explaining the cleaning procedure (a repeat of the wipe down with the sticky antiseptic wipes), handing me bags for my clothes, putting labels on everything. Pretty quickly, I was hooked up with heart monitors, an IV, and an oxygen monitor. Dr. L came in to discuss the mastectomy procedure and sign my right boob. "That one is part mine," she said.

Next, Dr. N came in to draw the plans on my skin. There was a lot of squishing and moving and sketching. We double- and triple-checked the plan, and she signed both boobs.

The anesthesiologist introduced himself and his nurse. He was quite pleasant and asked all the usual questions about whether I had ever had a bad reaction to anesthesia, how many surgeries I'd had, etcetera. He said he would monitor me the whole time and let my husband know I was doing well halfway through.

I was wheeled away to the OR and from down the hall I could hear my surgical team laughing and chitchatting. When I got there I said, "Sounds like you guys are having too much fun!"

They laughed and said they enjoyed working together, and that meant that I would have great care. This definitely put me at ease. Dr. L had her headlamp on, and I mentioned that it reminded me of Gonzo from the Muppets because it had a long bendy "nose" so she could adjust her light. That stuck and her medical assistant was off and running with the joke, saying it was definitely a good look for her. Dr. L smiled and said it was so she could get all the cancer out with her extra eyes, as well. Several more people came in, including the anesthesiologist, who chuckled at the reference to Gonzo, too. As I was transferred to the surgical table, I said, "Ooooohhh, you aren't going to have me awake much longer...." And I was out.

I was in surgery from 10:30 a.m. to 4:30 p.m. The surgery lasted this long due to a bleed that occurred in my left breast after Dr. N closed. She had to open it back up to find the bleed. Of course, by the time she opened it back up, it had stopped. Both surgeons were extremely happy with how things went.

I remember waking up in my own hospital room, but I don't remember how I got there. I remember my husband being there, but I'm not sure how he got there, either.

My husband reported that the first thing Dr. L said when she got out of surgery to report on my condition was tell him how much my breast weighed. He said he was a bit confused by that, but the surgeon knew I wanted to know. I wanted to know so that I could finish the Boob Weight Contest and grant the winner a bottle of wine and dinner (when I was up for it). My friend Melissa's husband won. He guessed 2.3 pounds. It actually weighed 1.3 pounds. Most people guessed way higher, including me.

In the hospital room, I gave the nurse my pain assessment on a scale from one to ten, and I answered with a three. They gave me ice chips, and I was left to snooze while they checked me every once in a while for vital signs. These puffy, squeezy things were attached to my legs to make sure that I didn't develop a blood clot. They inflated around one leg, then the other, then the other, then the other. All night. They made my legs sweaty and annoyed the heck out of me once my drugs wore off. "Seriously, someone turn these stupid things off," I bellowed.

I was encouraged to order something to eat that would be easy on my stomach. I chose applesauce and soup. Once it was presented to me, I needed anti-nausea medicine, stat. It took about twenty minutes for those drugs to kick in so I was able to breathe and concentrate on not throwing up. I got so close that I broke out into a sweat. But I prevailed against the puke, and I was able to keep all my pills and some applesauce down. Then I got another round of anti-nausea medication in my IV so I could keep everything down. My husband went home for a few hours to check on the grandparents and kids and to rest a bit.

It turned out that my husband couldn't sleep because I stopped answering his text messages, and so he actually drove back to the hospital at 4 a.m., but he couldn't get in. The hospital was closed to visitors! Dr. L mentioned that she hadn't worked with many patients who had a husband who supported her female patients in such a way by driving back to check on them. "I've never had a husband drive back in the middle of the night," she said. She also hinted that some of her patients' husbands were more concerned about the outcome of their wife's chest than their general wellbeing. My husband also purchased me a new pair of button-down pajamas that were comfortable and soft, and every shirt I wore for the six weeks after surgery would need to have buttons because I wasn't supposed to raise my arms over my head.

I had a surprisingly restful night. I didn't think I would be able to sleep, but the nurse said she heard me snoring, so I must have been asleep a few times. Of course, it's hard when a CODE GREY (which is apparently for a combative patient) comes over the all-hospital intercom, not to mention the constant checking on my vitals and encouragement to "void." (Why can't they just call it pee?)

By 7 a.m., I was awake and visited by both surgeons who peeked at the dressings and were (almost) giddy with the outcome. My reconstruction surgeon said, "I think they came out really pretty," which almost made me laugh. I had been so scared to look at them, fearing they would be bloodied and bandaged. They weren't at all and were quite small and perky!

On the other hand, there were the dreaded drains. I just couldn't prepare myself for them, and as I looked down to see the things, I realized I wouldn't ever get used to them. I had two drains, both hanging off my surgical bra on the right side. The drains entered my body in a small hole under my armpit next to my right breast. One drain tube settled in my body along the bottom of my right breast leading to the center of my chest. The other drain sat in the chest cavity of my right side. The holes in my body were covered by bandages, so that part wasn't gross to look at. It was the reddish, brownish liquid that collected in the two plastic bulbs hanging off a safety pin from my bra that bothered me. I had to unplug and squeeze the liquid out to measure it twice a day. Once the liquid hit 30 milliliters a day, the drain could be removed. I barely watched as they demonstrated the task for my husband, who was not queasy when it came to this type of thing. He would definitely be in charge of the drains.

My husband and I had breakfast (eggs and sausage—hubby had brought coffee earlier, thank god!!). It took a while to get dressed. I was discharged and a nice old man who volunteers at the hospital wheeled me out in a wheelchair to the car.

I knew my husband was happy to have me on my way home. My parents had taken the kids to miniature golf and out to lunch, and once they knew I was texting again, they sent me some photos. I knew my kids were being taken care of—spoiled, of course! The car ride home was uneventful, and I was surprised I could get my seat belt over the surgical bra and drains. Though, I did keep my hand against the strap all the way home. I kept repeating "This sucks," to myself. I probably said it out loud a few times, as well.

I was home. It was going to be hard.

My kids both seemed to understand that Mom needed rest and quiet. When I got home from the hospital, my daughter brought me a bowl full of strawberries and asked if we could share them. I was not hungry at all (side effects of the anesthesia I guessed), but I ate some and let her finish. She sat with me on our big chairs in the front window and watched the front yard for a bit before dinner. It was nice that she wanted to spend time with me. I think she was nervous. Frankly, so was I. It's hard to see your mom at Less Than, and I remember growing up, even though it was rare, that in the times my mom was in a Less Than state, it was disconcerting and unsettling.

My daughter reminded me four times in two days that I was not to move my arms too much. At dinner, she told me I shouldn't reach for my water and moved it closer to me. My girl. She repeatedly told me, "You'll do normal things once you are healed."

These kids will be OK. Now I'm worried about me. It seemed too easy. I was able to do things relatively well. I was up and around. I could get out of bed. I could walk. I didn't have much pain. There didn't seem to be much to recovery.

Andrea came over on Monday, four days after my surgery, and delivered me a cactus shaped like a penis (because she knows my humor) and chocolate-covered pretzels (because she knows what I love). We sat and chatted on the couch and then she took me for a walk down the street.

Later that day, I was sitting at the table waiting for my mom to prepare and serve dinner and I sighed and said, "My boobs itch!"

My dad replied, "Well don't itch them because Madonna would never do that! I don't know why I said that. It just seemed right."

I laughed so hard. I never thought how hard it would be for my dad—the father of a fiercely independent only child—to watch me go through this. And to be fair, I did talk a lot about my boobs that year, which I am sure made him uncomfortable.

A week after my surgery, my husband followed through on the idea of taking the kids away for a vacation. I felt relieved that I would have some quiet but remained wary about whether my kids would be OK without me—and if I would be OK without them. I'd never been without them until now.

> My kids are gone. It's—shockingly—the first time I have been without them for more than two nights since either one was born. My husband finally decided to take them to Las Vegas to meet his parents there. Las Vegas was one plane ride for everyone and hosted cheap hotels, especially last minute. I was sure the kids would melt, being Pacific Northwest born and raised, and it was the middle of summer in the desert. The trip ensured that everyone—except me, of course—still got a vacation. But the kids got a vacation with their dad and grandparents, and Mom got to rest.
>
> My concerns were two-fold, three-fold, infinity-fold. Because I am Mom and Mom knows what to do in every situation. Mom knows which kid is going to have issues peeing in public bathrooms; which kid is going to refuse to drink when prompted; which kid is going to test boundaries with bedtime; which kid is going to get homesick and how that is going to look with bad behavior. And it won't be obvious why and it won't be easy to overcome. But as a Mom, I know all the tricks. Who else is going to be Mom? I gave written and verbal instructions for what their health needs were, medications, etc., and everyone checked in with photos and updates.
>
> —*Blog post, August 1, 2019*

I thought I would have more time to miss them, but then I got sick. Really sick. The nausea was overwhelming. Friends were dropping off ginger candies, lemon and ginger tea, and anti-nausea bracelets. I used them all. It was like I was dying. Hot flashes climbed from my stomach to my head. The churning of my bowels and organs would not stop.

> My mother stood by my bed and fed me one Cheerio. Then another. Then another. Try dry toast. Gag.

One sip of water. I would fall asleep for a few minutes.

Another sip of water. Sleep. Overwhelming urge to rip my stomach out. No strength. Take one sip of water.

I just had to get the antibiotic pill in my body and make it stay. One more bit of Cheerio. Pill down. Breathe.

One Cheerio. One tiny sip of water. I am upright I cannot remember the last time I was able to open my eyes and not feel sick. So sick. One Cheerio. One tiny sip of water.

Suck on ginger.

One tiny sip of water.

It was the longest six hours of my life.

Skipping the Tylenol (which was all I took for pain) meant that the soreness all around my incisions and drains was back in full force. I needed to focus on getting those pills in and making them stay down.

Applesauce. One tiny sip of water. Pills. Down.

When I was able to sit upright, my mom said, "This was your dip. This is the worst day. It's done now. It gets better from here." Gosh I hope so.

—Blog post, August 1, 2019

I called my husband. I am not sure what I thought he could do, and in hindsight, I realized it wasn't the best idea. It turns out that it made him feel bad he wasn't there taking care of me, calling nurses, figuring out which drugs to take for what ailments and how high the risk for side effects was for each option. He asked why I called him and not my doctors. That wasn't helpful. But it was a good question. I just wanted him to tell me that it was going to be OK and that it was just a part of the recovery. He didn't do that. We don't have that type of relationship. There's not a lot of sugarcoating that goes on with us. There's a lot of realness.

I am not an easy patient. I am not an easy human. I do not give myself grace. It is who I am. Recovery forced me to reflect

a lot on this. I needed to hold myself to less vigorous expectations because I needed to recover. It was the only thing I needed
to be doing then. Not pointing out to my dad where he could
hang pictures (it had been on the list for a long time to get done);
not telling my mom which things could go in the Goodwill pile
(another thing that had been on the list for a while); not cleaning
out my closest because I wouldn't be able to wear most of the
tops I had. I was trying to find something to look forward to. I
was searching for the silver lining to the surgery, and I was genu-
inely excited to be rid of the DDDD bras. BRAS BE GONE!

About a week after surgery I had a morning post-op with my
mastectomy surgeon, who would give me my pathology results.
My mom and dad drove me to the office, and I checked in. Not
many minutes later, I was called back, leaving my mom to read
her book in the waiting room. My dad was in the lobby Starbucks
buying a Venti cappuccino and a newspaper.

A lovely nurse took my vitals and minutes later, Dr L walked
in. I could immediately sense that she was a bit on edge, but we
went through how recovery was going, how much liquid was
coming out of my drains, what my pain level was, and what I was
taking for pain.

She examined my breasts and remarked on how well they
were healing. The bruising found around both was subsiding and
looked good.

Then she briskly grabbed the pathology report. She first
went through the right breast, which was the full mastectomy
side with the implant. It came back clear. There was no remaining
DCIS in the tissue and there was no invasive cancer found. She
then said that the pathology found a very small amount of 1.8
millimeter DCIS in the tissue from the left breast.

Fuck. Wait.

Fuck.

Fuck.

Fuck.

I must have said it out loud because my surgeon said, "Yeah, that is what I said, too. Then I repeated it ten more times." She was not pleased, and I am guessing she was a bit surprised, too. She explained that it was too small an amount to show up on either a mammogram or an MRI, so all the testing that had been done on the left breast never would have shown it. The issue with this pathology report was that it didn't reveal the precise location of the DCIS. It's not accurate like a biopsy. They sampled tissue from the reconstruction but couldn't pinpoint where the 1.8 millimeter of DCIS was. It could be close to the breast tissue left in my body or it could be far from an edge, completely removed. So, we didn't know if there were clear margins.

> It was supposed to be a day of celebration. But instead, that other shoe dropped.
> I had so many party activities planned.
> I had so many awesome boob-related #hashtagideas planned for my friends.
>
> *—Blog post, August 3, 2019*

We discussed options—nothing new from what had been explained before.

(1) We could wait to see if any more DCIS showed up in a mammogram or MRI. That would be done every six months. Then I would have to wait to hear. Again, wait. That could potentially go on for fifty more years, or whenever you get to stop monitoring for breast cancer.

(2) We could do radiation. This would limit my options for later, as after radiation, skin does not heal as well, and many reconstruction surgeons hesitate to offer implants using your

own breast skin envelope as an option post radiation. This means I could never have "matching" boobs.

(3) I could take some sort of pill. I would have to schedule a meeting with an oncologist who could offer medication, (often taken for years) that inhibit hormones or something like that to stop DCIS from spreading. This sounded less like what I would want to do, but I didn't yet have the information to make an informed decision.

(4) I could have a mastectomy with implant. Matching boobs. Matching implants. More surgery. Well, honestly, this was the direction I was leaning, even without meeting with an oncologist to hear the third set of options. I had just gone through this, and it was not terrible. It was not fun, but I could do it again. Plus, it looks great. But what if I get it done and they don't find any more DCIS. Then I would have implants for, like, no reason.

> I asked my surgeon what she would do in my position. We all know doctors do not like to answer this question. But I think we have similar ideas on how to proceed and she seemed to answer honestly. She said that she would opt for the surgery route, and not just because she is a surgeon. I asked if she would suggest radiation for this particular situation and she answered: "I send a lot of people to radiation and believe in radiation as a treatment. I would have radiation myself. But not for this." That speaks volumes for me. I believe her. She told me that she called my reconstruction surgeon already (after she got the results the evening before) and they have already discussed options for me specifically. When I heard this, I felt such relief. I've only felt vulnerable one other time in my life—in Alaska trying to make the decision to climb down cliffs or go around another way—and it is a hard feeling for me. But I felt safe in the hands of these surgeons, who were clearly on the same page as I was. I felt like truly this

team of wonder women have my back (er, my breasts). We have already talked about getting on the calendar when its safe for me to have surgery again. My skin and body would need at least three months to recover from surgery.

The more I thought about it, the more it bothered me. If I hadn't had anything done to my left breast, no one would have found the DCIS until it showed up as a cloudy spot on my mammogram six months to a year later. Or never if it did not grow to become anything else. So, I wouldn't have known about it if I hadn't had my breast reduced to match the fake one. So, can I ignore it? If science wouldn't have found it, should I be worried about it? Can I pretend we didn't find it?

—Blog post, August 3, 2019

My surgeon agreed that this is the hardest part of this diagnosis. She suggested that I go see an oncologist to discuss the options for hormone therapy and radiation. But she also looked at me and said she would start looking at dates for surgery. She put her hand over my hand that was resting on my knee. She said, "We got this."

Upon further reflection, those rocks that were dislodged and rolled down the cliff as I was hiking down in Alaska were like the setbacks of my surgery—the first rock was my unclear margins with a mastectomy instead of reconstruction. The second rock was finding DCIS in my left breast. But each time in making treatment decisions in my cancer journey, I froze as the rock rolled by me, and I kept moving forward.

I texted my husband, who was at the Las Vegas airport returning home with my kids. He responded with, "Ugh. This sucks." Honestly, I wished he and the kids could have stayed away just one more day so I could start processing. I wasn't sure that I could greet them with smiles and hugs with this hanging over my head.

My mom and dad drove me from the appointment to buy some new bras. It was exactly what I *didn't* want to do. I didn't want to move forward. Not. One. Bit. But I did it. My mom was there. This is what moms do. They are there. Even though you don't want them to be. Because they are. And it was part of our original plan when we figured we would be done. So, we did it. We bought bras.

I couldn't try them on because I still had a drain, but I bought two front-clasping bras called "post-surgical" bras for when my drains came out. I don't remember the interactions with sales-people, but I also got a soft camisole for when I could lift my arms over my head again. It was a step in the direction of being done, but I also had an irrational feeling of resentment about these new bras, which would just hang in my closet and wait for me to be ready for them. They were just waiting. They didn't have to have more surgery.

I wanted to scream and punch things. Unfortunately, I couldn't do that due to recovery restrictions. It was the most intense amount of anger I have ever felt. This wasn't supposed to be what happened. This was seemingly against all the odds. I yelled at the whole universe. And my parents stood in the kitchen and let me scream.

I went upstairs to lie down. I never really rest, but I decided I could let my friends know what was up. I needed my village again. My friends had put this into perspective for me in the past, and I knew I could count on them again.

"Pathology results back. Right boob clear. Found DCIS in left boob."

Responses varied, but most of them included expletives and many exclamation points. Then the questions, "What next?"

I explained that I would have to see an oncologist/radiologist to decide next steps, and inevitably admitted that I would likely just have surgery. Immediately, GIFs of giant breasts and perky boobs came across my screen. I smiled. My friends knew me all too well. And even though I knew they were there, standing next to me even when they weren't physically there, I felt a sense of weakness overwhelm me. Even strong people have weak moments. And the weak moment arrived, and tears poured out of my eyes.

On the way to the meeting with the oncologist, I just shut down. I didn't want any more information. I didn't want to do this anymore. I was done—physically and mentally and emotionally. I understood that it was standard procedure to visit with an oncologist to talk about hormone blocking therapy to make sure that the other breast—which had been hiding at least 1.8 millimeter DCIS—did not grow any (more) DCIS. At this point, it seemed moot because I think in my heart, I had made my decision for surgery, but it was important to cross all the t's and dot all the i's.

The reception room of the oncology department was dismal. I thought to myself, "I am never coming back to sit in this room again." There were about equal numbers of men and women. I was the youngest person sitting there. There was a man with an inflamed red, puffy leg. There was another woman who just looked sad and ill. And there were the obvious chemotherapy patients wearing scarves around their heads. It was not the place I wanted to be. Still, I felt lucky that I was only there for a consult.

The doctor spent over an hour with us. She drew pictures of what a hormone blocker does to a cell (this was a revisit of college Biology class, so that was pretty easy to understand). It was also clear that she did these drawings for everyone she spoke with. I had an option of taking Tamoxifen, which is a hormone blocker that buffers the estrogen receptor to cells. Estrogen changes the cells so much they may turn into cancer. Tamoxifen blocks the estrogen from affecting the cell. Tamoxifen can also cause fatigue, hot flashes (which can be alleviated with a pill), mood swings (which can be alleviated with a pill), increased clotting issues, and uterine cancer. Basically, it comes down to taking this pill (with the possibility of two additional pills to decrease side effects) for five years, then once you are off it, you go through menopause.

As my husband put it, "Umm, that's like ten years of menopausal symptoms. Do I get a vote?"

Of course, I had to laugh at that—but only because I was not really considering taking the pill.

The doctor ran all the numbers for us. Here was the breakdown of recurrence of DCIS given the following scenarios:

1. Watching and waiting (mammograms/MRI every six months): 20% chance of recurrence in five years; 31% chance of recurrence in ten years.
2. Radiation only: 8% chance of recurrence in five years; 13% chance of recurrence in ten years.
3. Tamoxifen only: 10% chance of recurrence in five years; 16% chance of recurrence in ten years.
4. Radiation and Tamoxifen: 4% chance of recurrence in five years; 6% chance of recurrence in ten years.
5. Mastectomy: "cure" or 1% chance of recurrence in a lifetime; not enough breast tissue left to measure cells.

The doctor said I was extremely lucky to have the surgical team that I had working with me, and that she understood why I would have a mastectomy and implant, but that everyone's journey was their own.

One day later, I had my second drain taken out. It was awful. Not painful, just yucky. But it was finally gone. I spoke to my nurse about whether I needed to come back again, and she said that my healing was going really well, and I wouldn't need to be seen again unless I had a concern. She actually sent my reconstruction surgeon in to chat. We spoke about how disappointed we were to find the DCIS in the reduced breast. She presented all options for the next surgery (mastectomy with direct to implant) and we made a plan. She and my surgeon would discuss dates and get back to me.

With four more weeks of no laundry, dishwashing, or lifting more than ten pounds, I was starting to feel caged. I understood, though, that I couldn't move freely so that the scar tissue could form around the implant and stay in place. I was dedicated to following the instructions so that I could fully heal and get the best results. But I was seriously falling down a dark path with the next steps—not because I was scared, but because I was done. D. O. N. E.

I sat in my closet on the floor and typed "breast implants" into my search engine. I do not know why I did this. I think I wanted to hear that everything was going to be OK. I wanted to hear glowing examples of double mastectomy procedures with happy women skipping, braless, down the gold-paved paths of their jealousy-inducing lives. I did not read that. I spent the better part of several hours down a deep, dark rabbit hole of non-medical, highly emotional, very scary descriptions of breast implants. The internet showed me something called Breast Implant Illness (BII). Apparently, BII can cause general fatigue, brain fog, gastrointestinal issues, changes in taste, vertigo, pancreatitis, slow muscle recovery, frequent urination, dehydration, fibromyalgia, leaky gut syndrome, panic attacks, depression, heart palpitations, symptoms similar to Lyme disease, a host of autoimmune symptoms, fungal infections, night sweats, and the common cold. It was all there. BII caused everything. There are support groups. There are Facebook pages illuminating the dangerous and sickening consequences of implants. There are images of breasts, nipples, puffy legs, hair loss, doctor bills, and insurance statements.

And for two hours, I was convinced I already had it.

Because this is what happens when you do not know what else to do. You search it. You look for an answer where an answer does not necessarily reside. I sure did not get what I wanted down that rabbit hole.

So how did I get out of it? I did what I should have done in the first place, and I consulted a doctor I knew and trusted. I asked my breast cancer surgeon if she had heard of BII, and she replied, "You can find anything and everything on the internet, you know that."

I told her that I also looked up information through the American Cancer Society, the FDA, and the Mayo Clinic, which I thought of as reputable sources. She asked if I was put at ease by my searches.

"I would rather hear from you than the internet," I told her.

She replied that she had never seen a patient in all her years with anything that looked like Breast Implant Illness.

Onward!

My parents left after sixteen days because they saw that I was doing better, could drive, and, frankly, everyone was getting on everyone else's nerves. Before leaving, my parents set up my kids with a "recovery payment program" where they would pay each kid 50 cents for every task they did that I would normally do. This included making breakfast, loading the dishwasher, reaching into cupboards and the refrigerator, and laundry. It turns out they are quite capable kids! I knew this, but it was nice to see them step up. I was dying to know how long it would last. A week after my parents left (so, three weeks into my recovery), we were up to over $10 a kid. Not bad.

> See, the problem with being in the state I am in is that I look fine. I don't look sick. I am dressed and able to walk. It's just the singular use of my left arm that throws the kids. My son does not get at all that I can't
> use it. "It looks fine, Mom. You don't even have a Band-Aid." Truer words have never been spoken.
> But see this is where I just could not seem to move on. I still faced another surgery. I expected to be done by this point, yet it lingered. I also still had to recover. I just wanted to move on. But I kind of gave up. Because I still had people telling me that, "in 50 years, doctors won't even treat this type of cancer because it's not real cancer," and "I'm so sorry you still have cancer." How are these statements helpful? And they rolled around in my brain all day and all night. But I still got to have regular days like entertaining my kids and making sure they still have a "normal" summer, made progress on their summer extension workbooks, got excited about going back to school, ate too many popsicles, and had playdates.
> And as I sat and tried to relax and clear my head, it all came back. I still couldn't get my heart rate up so as not to increase fluid buildup, and I had to endure the creeping depression without the tools I normally had to combat it. I don't have any pants that fit due to the weight I gained since surgery. I didn't feel like going outside. But I had to have sunshine in order to feel better. It felt like a never-ending circle. But there I sat, halfway between depression and limbo. And there is where I would stay until what I was determined to call my Final Surgery.

> —*Blog post, August 12, 2019*

It was three weeks into my recovery, and I got the phone call to schedule a mastectomy with direct implant in December. It snuck up on me. Of course, I got the call when I was driving in the car with my kids, so I had to call her back. I was completely dumbstruck, unable to make a coherent decision. I hemmed and hawed for over three hours, asking my husband, parents, and all the friends within texting distance which date was best. I settled on December 19, 2019. But then I started worrying—was the surgery date too close to Christmas?

There was no right answer, but so many things to weigh: My parents insisted on being with us for the surgery to help with the kids and make sure I recovered well. If they came too early, they would be at my house for a month (and no one would survive that). I figured having my kids in school while I recovered was a good idea because it would give me quiet during the day. However, I didn't want Christmas to be ruined.

Maybe I couldn't decide because I just didn't want to do this again.

I called back and changed my surgery date to December 12. Then, my parents could stay two weeks and still be here for Christmas (which is our tradition), and they would not overstay their welcome. And I still had the kids in school for a week so that I could rest during the day.

Decision made.

Next?

> That is something that I have been having a ton of trouble with—moving on. Maybe it is because I have nothing to look forward to, at least not in the short term. I have another surgery to "look forward to." Though I have started thinking about it, I am scared to plan my "Cancer Free Party," in case I jinx it. I never

thought I would be a person who thought I could jinx anything, but cancer can alter your mind in so many ways. I want to be one of those people who believes so strongly that this is a Lump in the Road. But sometimes the reminder that I had cancer and still have cancer slams me down so hard I can hardly breathe.

Sometimes the only way I get through the day is by focusing on one thing. At that moment, I chose to look into my kids eyes every single time they speak to me. Because in that moment, that was what was going to get me through the day.

—Blog post, September 23, 2019

7

Limbo

October 2019

So, I needed a new bra. I was done wearing these hook-in-the-front, post-surgical, weird-line-making pieces of material. I also wanted to feel a bit normal again. Or start getting to a new normal. Before the next change.

Now, no one likes bra shopping, even with their own ta-tas. It's degrading to stand in front of a three-way mirror and examine the bulges over, under, and through the fabric, under your arm, or flowing out of the top of the cup. I knew what I wanted—something soft with hooks in the back. Something that is just there. I did not need a ton of support.

My friends were telling me to just go to Nordstrom, have them fit me, and get a few new things. So, I drove in traffic (oh my gosh, there was so much traffic) to Nordstrom and climbed to the third floor—lingerie. I swear the last time I was in Nordstrom was maybe five years prior. It's not my type of place. I do not feel comfortable there. I picked out four bras in several sizes and went to a dressing room. Most of them fit just fine. Some looked better than others. (I had only one nipple, so there were some logistical issues there, but I was pretty happy with what I found.) I went back out to pick some more and ran into a salesperson. (Do they have a better, more important-sounding title at Nordstrom? Probably.) I asked if she had any advice about a bra where the padding could be taken out of one side and left in the side with the nipple (these are the logistics I was referring to).

She said she would go find the bra-fitting woman who specialized in post-surgery and would send her right over. She congratulated me for making the huge step to come back to shopping. So, that made me feel somewhat better.

> A much younger woman came over and introduced herself to me and immediately asked if I knew that insurance paid for post-surgery bras. I said I was aware, but it didn't necessarily matter because I just wanted to walk out of the store with something that was comfortable. She told me that it seemed I should just come back and be fitted and make sure I had my prescription so they could bill my insurance. She kept using the word "augmentation" to describe my surgery, and I almost punched her in the face each time it oozed out of her mouth. You can't augment WHAT DOESN'T EXIST. Women who have mastectomies do not have anything to augment—except perhaps a chest cavity? That is why we call it reconstruction surgery. You are building up, not MAKING MORE BIGNESS and BETTERNESS. In every support group I have sat through or survivor I have spoken with, no one uses it. Its offensive to the survivor. This woman who is supposedly

trained in helping mastectomy patients should know this. FULL STOP. I'm guessing she gets paid pretty well, so, do your job better, woman.

—Blog post, October 4, 2019

I cried in the car leaving the mall. Because after all, anyone who has been through what I went through did need to feel like shit while trying to be comfortable. But at least I'd bought one bra for $38, which by the way, was half the price of any bra I had bought in the last twenty-five years due to my previous size. Whatever. I was happy with that and only that. I finally had one thing to wear that made me feel a bit "normal."

On top of all of this I found out that one of my family friends was diagnosed with cancer and is about to undergo radiation. I am surprised. And sad. And mad.

Oh also, one of my best friends in all of life, who does not live anywhere near me, has breast cancer. Caught early, but will still require surgery, radiation, possibly more. While her family history may have "predicted" a situation like this, there is no preparation you could ever do to hear the word "cancer" and be OK with it. Or not terrified. Or angry. Or sad. Or scared. I HATE being so far away. HATE HATE HATE. And now I know how she felt when I was going through my diagnosis and surgery... touché, universe, touché.

I called my mom to kind of vent about how I feel about these two cancer diagnoses. I pondered out loud to her about these people's medical journeys, and why, maybe, that one would have a Stage 0 cancer and still have to have radiation. She said, "Well, I fully expect that you are not done with your journey either. Your doctors have not gotten anything right yet, and at every step, there has been another thing come up. So, I expect you will have to have radiation after all."

And then all my words fell out: That is not helpful. You are not a doctor. Why would you say something like that? How does that help me live day to day until the next surgery? How am I not paralyzed by fear? How dare you. Fuck you.

I understand that as a mother, she felt helpless. She watched all this from afar. I understand that she comes from a different generation, where they didn't talk about every little thing, like we do. I understand because I am also a mom. Are you kidding me, Mom? And now I am mad and angry and mad and angry all over again. And I am stuck in a mad-angry cycle where I want to punch stuff. Also throw stuff. And scream.

And when I am done with all that punching, throwing and screaming, I have to prove her wrong. 100% wrong. And maybe she knows that this is who I am and it's a challenge. Honestly, I think that's the only way I can forgive her for her thoughts....

None of us should have to do this. I screamed, "Cure Fucking Cancer!!" Someone, please, fucking cure cancer.

—Blog post, October 4, 2019

I made it through six weeks of recovery. I thought I could be back to "normal" six weeks out of surgery because I was healthy and strong, I hardly took medications, and I was young. But I still couldn't reach anything above my head. My arms just wouldn't do it yet. It wasn't painful, but it was like the muscles and ligaments just didn't stretch that far anymore. I was surprised that no doctor prescribed physical therapy for me. I researched some stretches to do so I could feel some sort of progress. But none of it would be quick enough for me. I needed to get back to strong and healthy before we had to do it all over again in December. If I didn't, then I wouldn't have use of either of my arms at all. It felt like I was stuck in another limbo—a preparation limbo. It seemed hard to move on, but I was so desperate to have it behind me.

It was also still uncomfortable to sleep. Something was

always not right. The neck angle, the soreness of my arm all the way down, the tenderness of the incision sites, the zinging of the nerves that were starting to grow back. Nothing seemed to be normal, and I couldn't shake the feeling that I mentally and physically needed to get back to the gym, my regular schedule, and to seeing the people who lift me up with their smiles. I would definitely not be back to normal for a very, very long time. I guess I just needed to focus on being cancer-free.

This was the point in my journey I thought I could handle, but the waiting to do it all over again was emotionally taxing, which, in turn, proved to be very taxing physically. I found myself struggling with big and small things. I didn't feel like getting up in the morning. I dragged myself out of bed because I had kids who relied on me. It was the quiet times where I was not moving that were the worst. It was not anything in particular, and it was every little thing at the same time. When I played music, it was on repeat and it was loud. I was trying to drown out my thoughts.

The next Tuesday, October 8, I got myself to a support meeting in Seattle. It was next to impossible—being so far away and at Traffic Time. The honking, the screeching of tires, the rude drivers. The worry that I would be locked out of the building (it has normal office-hour-type hours). I got there, but barely.

I sat around the circle and recognized two people. I got to introduce myself quickly, and then the larger discussion about reconstruction and all the options available to new people were addressed. I sat across from a woman who had a double mastectomy for the same diagnoses as mine (DCIS—no chemo, no radiation). She had expanders. She was deciding between implants and a DIEP Flap Surgery (what I was originally looking into). Women asked questions, they answered questions, and all of a sudden, it hit me: If I had decided on the DIEP Flap Surgery (using your own stomach fat to make a breast), I would just be at the point in my recovery where I was able to move my arms, and I would be scheduling the left breast reduction. I wouldn't even know yet that there was DCIS in my left breast. In the weeks following a reduction, I would find out that DCIS was there, and I would then face the decision that I am currently thinking about. BUT because I had a deep tissue transplant, and I only have enough stomach fat for one breast, I would be forced to choose an implant. It was the very thing I was initially, months ago, determined to avoid. And though the surgeons would do their best to make them match, there is something very different about a tissue transplant and an implant in aesthetics. So, they would never really look similar.

MIND BLOWN.

One of the women at the support group told me that it looks like I made the right decision—she must have seen the look on my face as my brain processed everything. I was shocked I didn't think of that. I couldn't believe that it hadn't even occurred to me. I had made the decision and moved on. I didn't give it another thought—honestly, I didn't. I had just moved on.

My calendar popped up a reminder that I had a board meeting for PTSA. In this particular board meeting—remember, life doesn't stop for cancer—I gave up a fight I would normally take on. It was about something I felt pretty strongly about. But I didn't tell anyone how I felt. I didn't use reason and experience to make a strong argument for running a better program; for pointing out the missteps that we could address for the next year. I had prepared a whole list of issues to address. But it just sat in my notebook. I had never behaved this way before.

I watched as a friend and colleague tried to hold someone else at the meeting accountable. She was largely met with arguments of, "This is not the time or the place," from other board members. I seethed. But I let it go. I sat at the table and doodled things in my notebook, knowing full well that it was unlikely we would see this person—who had bitten off more than she could chew and failed to ask for help—again in any context at school. She would likely check out, and her name would just be on our board list for the rest of the year. She was done. I sat and listened to excuse after excuse, and lie after lie, and I thought to myself, "Why bother?"

As I walked home after the meeting, I asked myself why I let it go. I had spent so many weeks thinking about how to set this whole event/affair straight, how to make sure that it would not happen again, how to ensure that the right person was always sitting in the right position on the executive board. And I wanted to feel bad for not fighting. I wanted to feel like I had done wrong because I did not stand up for what I believed was right. But it turns out that I was tired of fighting for what cannot be changed. My body was tired of fighting. My mind was tired of being angry for things I couldn't control.

> Cancer messed with my head. I struggle so much about my diagnosis and treatment and plan of action that I felt helpless and couldn't control anything. I felt like I was being taken on a trip I didn't pack for. But I figured out I could control how I could approach things. I felt bad for not standing up for my colleague. She is my friend.
>
> I can control how I move forward. How I "right" the "wrongs." And how I can make something better out of something shitty. And that is one thing I learned from all

of this: pick your battles. You can only control your own reactions to shitty things.

—*Blog post, October 16, 2019*

It all started to wear on me. The little things—the things I used to take for granted—that should have been easy just weren't. I kept using "this was a hard year for me," as an excuse for when I randomly sat down to cry. I realized that I shouldn't need to use my Lump in the Road as an excuse for emotion, but it kept sneaking up on me. For example, after a long, brisk walk with my family at a local hiking spot, we returned home to get cleaned up before dinner. We all took warm showers, but by the time I got to sudsing up my hair, the hot water ran out. I jumped out of the shower, wrapped myself in a big, blue towel, and started wailing. I was cold. So cold. I was fully-body shivering with chattering teeth. I was cold to the core. And soapy. I just wanted a simple, hot shower. Did I not deserve a hot shower? And while this seemed like a small annoyance, it devastated me on multiple levels. I was still recovering from surgery, I was still reminded that cancer lived within me, and my surgical sites, though technically healed, were still tender and nerves were still growing back. It was just a shower.

And that's it, exactly. I just wanted a hot shower. Again, I had put my family ahead of me and made sure they were cleaned up and settled before dinner, before I took care of myself. And for that, I was granted cold water. It was the opposite of what I really needed. I needed something that should have been easy, to actually *be* easy. My takeaway from this one snapshot of life postsurgery, was that my journey with dealing with something as big as cancer hovered over me constantly, whispering to me in quiet moments that the easy things have to be easy. I was reaching my tipping point.

And then it snuck up on me. I knew it was coming. It was always knocking around in my brain. Always. But that didn't stop me from being utterly overwhelmed when the call came to schedule a pre-op appointment with my surgeon.

At the appointment, I knew exactly what to expect. I knew all the things that were going to happen. Blood pressure was great. Oxygen level was great. Temperature normal. I took off my clothes "from the waist up."

We discussed the next steps, which were basically the same as my first surgery: full mastectomy, with nipple sparing to be determined by my reconstruction surgeon. There were many variables to take into consideration with sparing a nipple, including Dr. N needing to use it as skin to make sure the left and right breasts would match. Saving a nipple has low risks, as the blood flow is sometimes not enough during recovery for the nipple to survive. I listened and nodded. I understood.

After examining the nodes under both armpits, doing a vigorous examination of my breasts and noting that healing was going really well, we discussed not going after the left lymph nodes as the amount of DCIS found (and taken) was so small that they did not expect to find anything invasive and didn't feel the risk to digging into lymph nodes was worth the possible side effects. (Some patients who have lymph nodes removed experience lymphedema, which is a swelling that develops in the hand, arm, or breast after mastectomy surgery or radiation. Side effects include swelling, tingling, and pain.)

She made sure that I understood that she would be following the reconstruction surgeon's directions for where to cut. Like Dr. L had said before, "I just color in between the lines." All the reconstruction decisions would be made by Dr. N, post-op and pathology results would be with Dr. L, but ultimately, reconstruction and aesthetics would be with Dr. N. It would be the same surgery as last time. I was feeling pretty at ease.

She asked if I had any second thoughts. I said no.

And then I began to think…

> No, still no. It was my decision to be on the conservative and safe side. I do not ever want to think about breast cancer again. I don't ever want to wake up and think, "is this the day my DCIS turns into invasive cancer?" I really do not have any second thoughts on my decision.
>
> —*Blog post, November 13, 2019*

"Can we just be done after this?" I asked.

"That's the plan!" Dr. L replied. I told her I was scared to plan a date for a Cancer-Free Party, and that if we keep prolonging it, my plans for one would get bigger and bigger and bigger until it was a complete blowout.

She smiled, laughed, and asked what I had planned and when it would be.

I said, "February, please!! When pathology comes back clear, and I am fully recovered."

She mentioned some hilarious guess that random hook ups due to fun music, champagne, and dancing could happen!

I truly love my surgeon. She is real. She is funny. She is human. She saves lives.

Before she left, she made sure that I knew my only job was to stay well during cold and flu season and said that she would see me in a month. I filled out more paperwork and got my antiseptic soap. I desperately hoped it would be the last time I had to see that soap.

The last pre-op appointment with Dr. N was during a week when the universe threw me a bunch of challenges. My son was attacked by a bully at school. Then I was attacked by a parent at school. Family drama entered stage left, and I rounded out the week with preparations for the holiday season. Because it turned out, once again, real life doesn't stop for cancer.

The drive to the city still sucked. Music on. Loud. So many cars. It saddened me that I no longer needed navigation help to get to the breast surgeon's office. It was still $9 to park for thirty minutes.

> I held so much love for my doctors and nurses. They know I just want it done. They know I am ready. They know I am a rule follower, and though it did drive me insane, I will do nothing for two weeks and no cardio or lifting for six weeks. Yes, I have my soap, yes, people will be in the house taking care of me. Yes, I still have pain meds left, yes, I still have nausea meds left.
>
> —*Blog post, November 22, 2019*

We double checked that we were on the same page with procedures. The plan was for a mastectomy with direct to implant. Same size and shape as the right side.

My doctor sighed after we went through the procedure basics again and said to me, "I told your story today. And it helped her." She had told someone that after I had a successful reconstruction, the smallest amount of DCIS was found, and we were back to planning another surgery.

> I didn't know what to say to that. I helped someone by having cancer. It's weird to be happy about that. It's like the universe is pulling me in two directions. I would rather not have had the opportunity to help someone with this. But since I have to walk over this Lump in the Road, I may as well have helped someone.

I have been thinking so much about my *story* lately. I started writing again. While I am not a writer, I write. It does not mean anything will come of it. Maybe something "should" though. I have "Rewrite the Story" from the television show *Smash* in my head constantly lately. It is about how someone can start over after feeling so lost. It's a song about renewal and rewriting one's story.

What is it that I want to rewrite? Well, I sure as hell would love to be able to say I have never had cancer. I will take being able to say I am cancer-free in twenty days, though. I would really like to have a party. I would really like to stop being faced with the daily grind on top of having cancer. I would like to celebrate something big. Some people do not realize that every single day of my life I think about cancer. I struggle to find a bright spot among life's little things. Arguing about tiny things are literally not worth it to me. On the tip of my brain, I am still waiting for the cancer to get out and not come back ever. It is that simple. Tee minus twenty days until surgery.

—*Blog post, November 22, 2019*

And then the calls came. Two Fridays before surgery, I received three phone calls, all trying to schedule a radiation consult with me. With the first call, I calmly explained that I would not be needing radiation treatment, so please just take me off the list. The scheduler was a bit disappointed that I did not want to follow my doctor's orders that were on a screen in front of her. She hung up and said she would put a note in my chart that I refused a consultation.

Two hours later, I got another call from the same office, this time a different scheduler, trying to schedule a radiation consult for two-to-four weeks post-surgery. I less calmly explained that I would not be needing radiation as there would be no boob tissue to radiate.

The woman snapped back that she was not a nurse and was just following the doctor's orders.

I even less calmly explained that I understood that my doctor would NOT be recommending radiation, and besides, I already had a consult with the very doctors she was trying to schedule me with.

After she told me again to just make an appointment, I asked her to read from my chart the request for an appointment, which she did.

It was from my doctor's nurse, and it sure seemed like I would need radiation. I told her that I would not be making an appointment and I would call my nurses to double check.

I hung up on her. I was not sorry.

> Here is the deal. This is cancer we are talking about. And it's an office that deals with cancer patients. Every single office person who calls a patient has to realize the patient has cancer. Whatever stage, whatever part of their journey. You don't get to tell people what they need to do. You don't get to change the course of their journey for them. You have to realize that the mental capacity of a human with cancer is tenuous at best. And you cannot throw them a curve ball. It will ruin them.
>
> It ruined me.
>
> I felt like I handled most things up until that moment pretty well. This one series of phone calls wrecked me. I was counting down the days until I get pathology back. It will forever be a date in my mind—December 20. I am scared to hope that I am cancer-free, which is ridiculous because I should have hope. But given my journey so far, with the things that should have gone my way running the opposite direction, I was scared to hope.
>
> So, don't tell me now I need radiation, when my doctor told me I would be done after this.
>
> —*Blog post, December 10, 2019*

I turned to what I normally do when I can't face the unknown. I ran. I ran until my body wouldn't let me. I called and texted my village to cry, complain, bitch, yap, and scream, and then I sat in a puddle of tears, feeling completely empty. I felt like I didn't have any more emotions in me to feel. I felt like I could not have one more deviation from the plan. I couldn't face one more setback.

I had called my nurse before I ran and left a message. Three hours later she returned the phone call, and before I even confirmed it was me on the other end, she said, "Kate, I am so sorry. That message is automated, and you should not have received a phone call to make a radiation consult appointment." She said that 90% of people from her office are referred to a doctor for radiation consultation, so it is an automatic system.

None of that could be taken back. None of the emotions could be put back in the bottle. None of the energy expended could be reclaimed. But it was time to get back on track.

It was two days until surgery, and I was hoping so badly for it to be the last. I still had to make sure all the holiday preparations were in place so my kids' Christmas wouldn't be tainted by cancer. I wasn't feeling particularly Christmassy, and it was frankly exhausting putting up a strong, happy front for the people around me.

I had been apologizing a lot.

My friend Brandy called me out on this. She owns a local painting business, and I had been painting with her for months through my treatments because it brought me great relaxation and distraction. She is fun and real, and she was going to lead a painting class of a landscape of my choice for my Cancer-Free Party. There would be champagne, painting, snacks, and laughter, all to celebrate me being cancer-free! But then, I found myself apologizing to her because I wasn't sure I was going to schedule a big party yet. I told her that I did not want to jinx my pathology coming back by scheduling an event celebrating that I was cancer-free. So, I said I was sorry.

She said, "Did you just apologize to me for not being able to control cancer?"

Yes, I did.

Because surgery was on December 12, we were attempting to cram all the holiday activities (lights up, house decorating, holiday parties, tree cutting and trimming) into two weeks. It was incredibly stressful. I apologized profusely to my husband that had to find another tree farm place to visit (because of constraints of our schedule and the tree farm's), and he said to stop apologizing.

Why, though? Why couldn't I apologize?

I felt sorry that I had to do this, not for myself (though I can absolutely understand how people who are diagnosed feel sorry for themselves). I felt sorry the people around me had to rearrange their schedules. That my kids wouldn't have the normal Christmas things this year (though they didn't know that yet). That my friends had one more person to worry about. That my parents had to slog through mountain passes and rearrange their schedules and worry about me.

But cancer didn't apologize to me.

Surgery rolled around, and this time, it was an 11:30 a.m. check-in for a 12:30 p.m. surgery. I was able to walk my kids to school and see some people before surgery. My parents walked with me, and I think they were overwhelmed by the amount of hugs and well wishes I got. I hadn't had food for over eighteen hours by the time we left for the hospital, so I was hangry.

At the hospital, we walked past the same piano playing by itself, through the same hallway to the surgery reception, and spoke to the same happy receptionists. I answered all the same questions as before, and when they asked if I had any questions, I replied, "This is the third time I've been here, so I am all good."

My husband wasn't even checking in with me. He was grabbing a coffee and letting me get settled with my antiseptic wipe down, vitals, heart-rate monitor, and IV before coming back for the surgeons' visit.

Then the anesthesiologist and his nurse stopped by and asked if we had any questions. My husband asked routine questions he likely already knew the answers to, and the doctor left. Dr. L swung by, followed by Dr. N. They missed each other by minutes. Dr. N explained that she might put a substance called AlloDerm in with the implant in case the breast wanted to fall over to the side. Apparently, it is quite common with implants, and it is a substance like collagen, so it wouldn't be expelled by your body. This was a very last-minute decision, and I had trouble processing it, not because I did not want to do it—I didn't want to do any of this—but because I just wasn't expecting it.

By then, I cannot explain how cranky and impatient I was to just get under the knife. The surgical room was backed up, due to it being December with a packed surgery schedule for insurance reasons. It was past 1:45 p.m. when the nurse finally wheeled me into the OR. His name was Charlie, and he was jovial and chatty. He was the only one in the OR prepping it. I saw the anesthesiologist briefly, and then I remember nothing.

I woke up in the recovery room, and I clearly remember thinking there were too many people around me, everyone protected with curtains, but it almost seemed like we were all lined up. One of the nurses said, "Yes, call him, his wife is awake." And then my husband was by my side. We waited for a long time in recovery, and the nurse was getting frustrated with there not being a room available upstairs, so he just started wheeling me up and mentioned that a patient on their way up was a guarantee for a room being ready. The hospital was packed.

I was pretty comfortable with the pain, but I ended up throwing up from the nausea. No one else seemed fazed. Eventually, applesauce, crackers, and pudding showed up. It was too late to eat dinner, and I didn't feel like it anyway. This time around, I was super drowsy and just wanted to sleep. My husband left to go home after I assured him I really just wanted to sleep.

I slept well for about two hours, and then I was wide awake in the middle of the night, so I watched two Hallmark movies. I slept really well for almost two hours in the morning. My doctors all came in and said they were really happy. We chatted more about things other than my boob, so that was encouraging. My cancer surgeon said, "Are you glad to be done?" She was expecting a clear pathology report and said she would call if it came early.

The night in the hospital seemed to fly by this time, compared to the last time. We didn't even have time to order breakfast.

Once home, I was overwhelmed by the things I had to do: Christmas preparations, school deadlines, etcetera. I was not in a ton of pain, in fact it was quite manageable, so I had trouble taking it easy. My mom reminded me three times that morning to stop moving my arm. I taped my left elbow to my side and promised myself to stop moving it, because for long-term recovery, I needed to take it easy.

8

You Have a Message

December 16, 2019

It had been the normal schedule of recovery—walking slowly, drinking water, taking meds on time. It was hard to take it easy because it was the holiday season and there was always so much going on. Occasionally, my phone would beep with an email saying that I had a message in MyChart, the online platform my doctors used to communicate appointment reminders, bills due, and test results. Each time, my heart skipped a beat, wondering if it was the results I had been waiting ten months for. Was it the pathology report?

Beep. Not this time. It's only a reminder for a post-op appointment.

Beep. Not this time. It's a reminder to pay a bill.

Then there it was: *Beep*. You have a test result.

My parents had just left to pick my kids up from school. And there in my inbox, after the usual *beep*, was an automated email from MyChart.

<You have a test result available in MyChart.>

Already?! I had already gotten the glucose panel, the hemoglobin, and whatever the heck else they test for post-surgery. It wasn't December 20 yet. That was the date I was expecting to get news.

I sat down to log on from my phone. It was a huge pain to do, as my fingers are too big to type the password in after scrolling to the side. But I had done it a hundred times before.

Surgery pathology report. There it was.

Breathe.

Read.

Breathe.

Read.

Breathe.

Read.

I reread everything again because my brain could comprehend nothing.

Again.

Again.

<Benign breast tissue consistent with central duct region origin.>

<No in situ or invasive carcinoma identified.>

And I panicked.

Cried and panicked.

I waved my hands in the air around my face and I said, "That's it. That's it. It's over. I am done."

I said it over and over like someone in the empty room needed to hear it. I said it quietly, then much louder. Then I said it again. And I kept crying. It was an emotion I don't think I have ever felt before. It was a relief combined with gratitude, combined with disbelief, and a sense of emptiness. But it started so deeply in my heart that I couldn't express it in words. I didn't know whom to thank first. I almost couldn't believe it.

It wasn't until hours later—and after reading the report many more times—that I realized my doctor had written a note at the top of the report: <Finally a completely benign pathology report. It's time to party!!!—Dr. L.>

> At every step of this journey, I felt like I had the most competent, understanding, and realistic team of surgeons and medical staff. I have never felt like my doctors did not have my back. That they weren't standing right next to me, ready to catch me if I fell over. If I stumbled, tripped. And I feel like we metaphorically did all of that. To have a surgeon who has been alongside me, respecting me, swearing with me, and celebrating with me the whole way is a blessing.
>
> I have not ever believed in luck or blessings, but I believe in strength and gratitude. And I have both. And so does my surgeon. Both of my surgeons, actually. And I have so much respect for them and appreciation for the respect they have shown me on every step of this journey.
>
> But the journey isn't over. It's time to recover. It's time to celebrate.
>
> *—Blog post, December 17, 2019*

It felt like the rush that I had gotten at the bottom of that cliff in Alaska, a sense of relief packed with heart-racing adrenaline. I faced a challenge. I was finally able to look back up at that cliff knowing I conquered it.

Two days after I received the MyChart message, I had a post-op with my ARPN, since my surgeon was on vacation for the holiday season. The nurse took my vitals and told me to, "put the robe on from the waist up, tie in the front" an instruction I must've heard a hundred times by then.

I was up on the table swinging my legs back and forth, wondering what we would really do at this appointment. It was still too early to take my drains out. Heidi came in an asked how I was and how the recovery was going. She asked if I had seen Dr. N and what she thought of recovery this time around. She asked me how I was *actually* doing with all "this."

I took a deep breath and started talking about my frustration with how I am approached by so many people who have opinions about my condition and my diagnosis and my choices. How some people do not see DCIS as real cancer, and how although I had not had many people question my choices, there were a few raised eyebrows directed at me regarding how I chose to treat DCIS.

We spoke about mutual experiences where people would tell us they had a cure for cancer, whether it was a certain type of leaf you can put in tea, or the thought that cancer can be caused by stress and the inability to slow down. Heidi had been doing her job for years, and she noted that so many people stand on a soapbox and tell you their strong opinions about what they would do, but until they are faced with making decisions about their own bodies and their own lives, it isn't really fair to offer those opinions.

I mentioned that it was hard to get over to the support group in Seattle, and how, even though there seemed to be so many people in our area (east of Seattle) that are diagnosed with cancer, there seemed to be a lack of mediated support groups.

She mentioned that I could call and speak with the hospital's social worker about the need to start a group at the hospital, as Heidi knew several patients who would be willing to participate. I told her how it had really helped me to write down my journey in a blog. She mentioned that she read my blog.

I held my breath.

She said that she found my blog honest and thought that it filled a void in resources for so many women they see in their cancer clinics. She thought that if I were to make my journey public, it could be a resource for many women who have a DCIS diagnosis. And she said, "While I can't ask you to write a book, your voice would be so helpful to the women who are going through this and have no one to look to for the real journey." She said there are not many sources her patients can go to that are "real" and "raw" and "practical."

I was somewhat speechless, and I may have said something along the lines of being happy to help other people.

She smiled and stood up. Before she left, I asked her if she wanted to see my sutures. She said no, and that she hoped I had a good Christmas, given the circumstances. She wished me well.

Although that conversation left me feeling hopeful and positive, the recovery process can be full of setbacks and disappointment. I was disappointed that I still had eight milliliters to go before my drain could come out. And being the Christmas holiday, no office was open until December 27th, so I had to wait until then anyway. It didn't hurt, but it was annoying to have something hanging off my body, and it made me feel like I was sick. It was a barrier to getting back to normal.

So was having my parents living with us. My mother is quite adept at doing dishes, laundry, and vacuuming, which was very helpful. But I was still making my own coffee and pouring my own cereal. My kids were a wreck, with the usual holiday craziness and lack of listening. Consequences given were ignored, and it felt like they disrespected every single thing I said.

> It was finally Christmas and I hated it. I was in a bad mood. I hated the holidays and everything they stood for. I wasn't feeling very giving. I wasn't enjoying my family or kids. And worst of all, I didn't feel bad about it. I wanted to be left alone. I didn't want to hear anything. I didn't want to hear kids laugh or scream with delight. I didn't want to answer questions about presents or anything about Christmas cookies this year. I wanted absolute silence. I wanted to wake up when my body said to wake up. I wanted to go to sleep when my body said to. I didn't want to have to worry about any one thing, any human being, or anyone's feelings.
>
> I wanted to run away.
>
> I should've been thankful that the sun was out, as it had been pouring for days. I should've been thankful that I was cancer-free, though it hadn't quite sunk in and I hadn't had a chance to process it.
>
> —*Blog post, December 24, 2019*

And through all of this, I had to continue like I didn't just get a new lease on life, like I didn't just go through ten months of hell and the unknown on emotional roller coaster. I had to pretend that it was a regular holiday and that regular things were going to happen.

> And then there is the thing about yeast infections in your armpit. Apparently, it is a thing. And I got one Because I followed the directions of my doctors, not lifting my arm at all. Of course, I need one more thing to make me feel like I will never get back to normalcy.
>
> Also I could braid my leg hair. It was the first time since I spent 30 days backpacking in Alaska that my leg hair was so long I could pet it. Because moving my arms like that to shave is also not allowed, so it couldn't

be a priority when trying to clean myself up. It was
kind of amazing how trying to return to normal was
seemingly impossible when I couldn't do normal things,
small things, like shaving legs. I knew I would get there
eventually, but it was just another Lump in the Road to
recovery.

—*Blog post, December 30, 2019*

I finally got my drain out, thankfully, after Christmas and
before a weekend. I couldn't get an appointment with my regular
nurse, so I went across the hall to a different nurse. I was, apparently, her fifth drain removal of the day. She was a nice nurse,
who asked me a bunch of questions: How was Christmas? How
many milliliters was I getting out of the drain? Had I had a drain
before? She was pleased that it would not be my first drain pull
(it's literally what they call it, and is a most accurate term) but
said she would explain everything as she was doing it so I would
be prepared. She took the tape off very carefully—my skin really
likes to hold onto tape. She swabbed the area and cut the one
stitch that held the plastic tube in the side of my body, under my
armpit. She asked me to take a big deep breath in and…

Zzzzzzzzziiiipppppppp!

DONE.

It did not really make a noise. And I couldn't really feel it.
But it was uncomfortable afterward, mostly because I knew she'd
pulled something out of my body. She had to hold a gauze there
for a few minutes because the drainage was still leaking out a bit
(yeah, it's gross), and she mentioned that I might have to change
the bandage, but that the hole would close in about forty-eight
hours (yeah, super gross).

She congratulated me on following all the directions and
wished me a speedy recovery. I appreciated her willingness to

listen to me chat away. (I really get nervous when it comes to the drain—it's just one of those really icky things for me.)

And I left. My dad drove me back home. I felt like I needed to celebrate, but also, I felt like I still had a long road ahead of me. I still had at least one more post-op appointment, and the next four weeks of not moving my left arm.

> Yes, I was finally cancer-free. But still... a long road to recovery. It was still hard because even though I am cancer-free, it's a challenge to process everything as being over. Because I don't think it is. I don't think that people who have been through a cancer diagnosis (at whatever stage) are ever really DONE with having that diagnosis; we don't ever leave behind that pounding in the chest of hearing the words "It's cancer"; the feeling of dread in wondering if it's around the corner again; the guilt of not celebrating every second we are cancer-free; the inability to put into words how it has changed us.
>
> —*Blog post, December 30, 2019*

This wasn't necessarily an end for me. In fact, after hearing Heidi, my ARPN, speak about my blog and how it could help people, I began toying with the idea of making the blog into a book.

That same afternoon, a friend who had a similar diagnosis but a very different journey, pulled me aside and, with tears in her eyes, and said that she read my blog and it took her back to her own diagnosis. Because what I wrote was so real. That she said she is not the type to go to support groups, and that she would've liked to read something like this when she went through her journey. She was reliving the emotions I put on paper as her own.

She said she had been bouncing around life, not thinking anything like cancer could happen to her. It's not in her family. She didn't expect it. Especially, in her case, being so young.

I allowed her to feel, to vent, to emote and relive it. Because that's what we do as survivors. The fear and the shock, the realness, it is overwhelming and hard to put into words, but it makes your heart feel deeper. It's a part of the journey. And sometimes it comes back as waves.

I can honestly say I was deeply affected by this. Throughout this whole Lump in the Road, I have been saying to myself, "If me going through this and writing about this helps just one person... maybe it's worth it." And maybe that's why this happened. I do not believe in destiny, and I likely won't ever believe in fate, but if something good can come out of something bad, who am I to stop it?

—Blog post, December 30, 2019

.

9

The End?

January 2020

I was driving to Seattle for my very last post-op meeting with my reconstruction surgeon, Dr. N. The drive in the torrential downpour was nothing new. I turned my playlist up to window-shaking decibels and merged onto the highway. Just as I was exiting at the 520 bridge for Lake Washington Boulevard, I saw a rainbow. It seemed to end right at my doctor's office.

I took it as a sign that there was a chance that this journey, with a Lump in the Road along the way, was at its end.

I pulled onto the streets that by now I knew by heart. I turned left into the Nordstrom Tower, drove up to the ticket machine and pushed the "ticket here" icon on the screen. I zipped the car up to the third floor, so I had to take only one elevator to floor sixteen. I looked out from the top floor. It was a rainy and dreary view.

The front desk staff greeted me by name. I said hi, and we chatted about the cost of tolls over the bridges.

I was called immediately back and given a warm gown. No one even said to make sure the ties were in the front anymore. I stripped down on top and put on the gown. Not one minute later, Dr. N knocked and popped her head in.

She asked how I was.

"Good," I said.

She asked how I was feeling about everything.

I said, "I am feeling good, especially now that it's all over. I think they look fine."

After feeling around the implants a bit, she said they were sitting well. The only other things that could be done/altered were adding a nipple to my right breast and maybe doing a fat graft to add a bit of roundness to the upper right breast.

"Would you consider it?"

"Nope."

She has always been beyond respectful and has never pressed any issue. The nipple topic was dropped.

I had heard several things about monitoring my breasts after surgery. I asked about this and Dr. N said I did not need to have an MRI every few years because the implants are saline and won't cause any ill effects if they leak. And I will know if that happens because I will deflate. I also asked about a prescription for a bra since I needed to be properly fitted for an expensive post mastectomy bra, though I was not looking forward to another trip to the bra fitters.

She grabbed her camera and pulled down the black screen for after photos. We chatted about the party I was planning while she took photos. I also mentioned I would be writing a book, and she said, "Yes! You totally should!"

We chatted a bit more, and she said if I ever needed anything or changed my mind, to come see her. She asked to see photos from my party. She told me about an amazing bag decorated with artsy breasts that I could carry my book in once it was published.

I walked out. The hallway was empty. I pushed the elevator button. *Ding.* I got in and went down to floor three.

WAIT.

I forgot my prescription! I stopped in my tracks, "Do I really need it?" I hesitated then walked back to the elevators. Up to the sixteenth floor.

I explained at the front desk that I forgot the prescription for a bra, and they sent me to Tifni, the office manager who took care of scheduling between various offices and insurance. I said it was no rush, but if she could just forward it to me or put it in MyChart that would be great. We ended up chatting about the movies our kids watch.

The prescription was in my inbox before I got home, along with a link to another movie she thought my kids would like. There are no words for that kind of service. It's not even really service. It's a sisterhood. It's a village. It's a support group. It's just kindness and realness. It's understanding that we are all humans together in this journey—with bumps in the road, big or small.

I got back to my car and turned the music up again. I paid my money and got back to the highway. Traffic was backed up for miles. Once on the bridge, it opened up, and I started to breathe. I wondered when it would hit me that it's over. Like, no more. I get to move on. This was the moment I was desperately waiting for.

I drove by some construction on the left, and then I sucked air in. And then it was hard to catch my breath and the tears ran down my face. My chin quivered and I knew it was not going to be pretty. I kept driving and crying.

But back to actual reality. After six weeks of not being able to do things, what was the first thing I did? I went to the grocery store. Because I was finally allowed to lift the bags. And I bought an ice cream cake and champagne.

Because.

Because we celebrate the big and small.

Because life is too short, and we don't know what's coming.

Because it creeps back in.

My husband texted me that not having cancer is something to be happy about. Well, of course it is. But that's not it. I would always have a reminder that I went through this journey. From listening to other women's stories, I understood that they became less frequent and there would be more time in between each one, but we have a reminder emblazoned on our chests. Literally. My boobs, as pretty and perky as they may be, are a constant reminder that I had a hard thing to deal with. And yes, I came out of it stronger with a more powerful voice, but the reminder is there. Every single day. But it would not define me.

Ten months after my diagnosis, I was having trouble processing the whole year. I drove and thought to myself, "Just ten months ago, everything was Before Cancer. It was Regular Life." Then an influx of emotions would overwhelm me.

It kept me awake, and I felt unable to process what I had been through. After it all, now that I was cancer-free and I was planning a huge party, nothing was coming naturally to me. I felt like I was trying too hard to make it happen, to feel like I could celebrate.

I watched myself interact all year—on Facebook, in my daily interactions. And it was all about life going on around me despite my cancer diagnosis. I never felt like I could post the tumultuous journey on social media—not for any reason other than I just didn't want to share. I had my village, my support group, and I did not feel the need to advertise that I faced a Lump in the Road. But if I had, here is what I would've written:

> This year has sucked. It has been real. It has been raw. I couldn't wait for it to be over. Not because it was 2019. Because I had cancer. It's not something I ever expected to have to deal with—and that's exactly what I did. I dealt with it. I didn't wallow, I didn't ask for help, I ran into it head on. And I won. But as I think back to last year, it hits me that I didn't ever post about it because life goes on. It kept going on. Life around me never stopped. And I didn't want it to. Because if it did, I wouldn't be able to move on or move forward.

And in thinking back about the past year, I realized that it would be a while before I could trust that something else wouldn't go wrong. But as of January 8, 2020, my reconstruction nurse said all healing looked excellent, my breasts were pretty, and the pain I felt under my arm was absolutely normal inflammation from where they pulled the drain.

But then it would all sink in again. Depression. It made almost no sense that I would feel depressed. Almost none. But when I sat in my office, checked emails, or bought something from Amazon, I was gloomy—not the kind of gloomy that I couldn't get myself out of eventually. Just not in that moment. I was content that I recognized that I was sad and depressed.

There was also just less brain noise after everything I'd been through. When I sat in a silent room—which was quite rare with having two kids— I was no longer running through the what-if's and the when's of the diagnosis and ensuing journey. Instead I was back to the running list of a mom who has too many things to get done to make sure her and her family's lives are fulfilled. Grocery list updated, rain boots to replace the ones a kid just outgrew yesterday ordered from Amazon, a PTSA email answered, an email to a teacher sent, a bill paid, a check written, insurance payment double-checked… it was all a never-ending hum that I was so grateful to be back to, but I also heard the silence. And the silence was the void that reminded me that I'd been through the journey and I didn't have that worry right now, though the worry never went away completely. The thought that I was just living my life (bouncing around and being busy) and did not expect this cancer diagnosis and having it blindside me was a wake-up call.

Like a wake-up call that another something is around the corner.

> And maybe that's what this episode of depression was. It was the anticipation of waiting. It's the wanting to plan a celebration and wanting to celebrate and wanting to be able to breathe but not being able to out of the fear of something else.
>
> And that makes cancer win.
>
> I know cancer is not a thing that can plan, that can decide to choose someone else. It's a biological fact. It doesn't have a life of its own. It doesn't have free will. But in the case of being rid of it forever, I now think it has the upper hand. Because I wasn't supposed to get it—I wasn't predisposed. No one in my family has died of cancer that wasn't caused by something (like smoking). So, I didn't expect it.
>
> Now I don't know what to expect. And maybe it's that I thought I wouldn't have this fear. That I would think I was completely done with breast cancer. Because I have no breast left, so how could I have breast cancer again? It's the fear of being blindsided again that wins.

Being blindsided by something that wasn't supposed to happen.

But I guess that's how it's always supposed to be—it's the definition of blindsided. It's unexpected.

The question is how to move through this—not move ON, like I am leaving something behind. Because this journey is not something I can leave behind. It is something that comes with me, every day, and hides somewhere. It is my job to figure out how to learn to live with it and be content, happy, and joyous. And for right now, that has to be enough.

—Blog post, January 15, 2020

I survived the worst, but I had to admit I was not grateful every second; and I felt guilt that I didn't have complete and utter joy all the time.

In those moments I realized that what changed most about myself and what surprised me most about this year were one and the same: I was strong when I didn't have to be. It was a long ten months from diagnosis, to surgery, to having my last post-op appointment. And looking back, I felt like I didn't scream enough. Or cry enough. Or wallow enough. Because there really is not any more appropriate time to do those things than when you're diagnosed with cancer—of any kind.

I think that after my initial, gut-wrenching collapse to the ground, there were only two other moments of complete weakness: once on the floor of my closet, feeling really sorry for myself that I was forced to make all these decisions that were not a part of my life plan; and another time when I just stood in my living room screaming that it wasn't fair that I had cancer.

Three times I lost my shit. In ten months.

In retrospect, I feel like I should've given myself more chances to collapse. And my friends reminded me that it was OK to lose it. But I didn't. I just kept going. Because my kids and their lives wrapped around me, distracting me, but also reminding me it was important to keep going. And honestly, life kept going on around me. It couldn't stop.

My friend Sam mentioned that I was allowed to be depressed and sit on a couch all day and wallow. She even suggested it. But there I was, at pickup, at drop-off, at swim lessons, at the gym. Because why would I wallow? I always wanted to make decisions and get through. Move on.

And because I have an amazing friend, Kate (who lives too far away), who keeps me motivated and keeps me on track. I have been able to write about the journey and my process. And it was through this that I could share my actual feelings about things, not out loud, but in a raw way, and I feel that I found my voice. And through my voice I found strength.

Then, just when you think you have had a chance to catch your breath, uncertainty is right there again, around the corner. It happened sooner than I thought. I always knew that I would have to think about cancer, but I thought I could catch a break for a little while.

My husband was helping me take a splinter I could barely see out of my toe, and he glanced at my ankle and said, "Wow, that looks cancerous. You need to have that looked at."

I just stared at him. My chin quivered. Tears welled in my eyes and flowed down my face. He looked away. He didn't get it. I screamed out loud, "Why would you even say that to me?!"

I had been watching the smeary freckle on the side of my ankle for years. It didn't really change, until this past year, when it grew a tiny, pinhead-sized dot of dark, dark brown. I promised myself I would get around to it, but I just didn't want to see another doctor. I didn't want to drive to the hospital. I didn't want to walk up to the receptionist and give my name and date of birth. I didn't want to wait in another waiting room. I didn't want to have my vitals taken. I wanted none of it. Medical fatigue.

I just *had* cancer. I can't have it again, right?

NO! I am done with it.

I hadn't begun to heal emotionally, though physically I was doing quite well. Emotionally I was scarred.

But I did it. I made an appointment to see my doctor, whom I love, and who hadn't seen me since she did my annual checkup and hadn't spoken to me since she gave me the news that I had DCIS.

> I drove to the hospital without thinking, like so many times I have done it this year. About a block away from the right-hand turn into the street the hospital is on, tears streamed down my face. My stomach dropped. I let the tears fall. I don't need to hide them anymore. I am not embarrassed by them falling. It is not a sign of weakness but a sign of weariness. My soul was weary from worry. It has been a year almost to the day that I had my first annual (and last) mammogram, and I should've predicted these feelings, but I couldn't predict their intensity. It creeps in. I wish so hard that these anxious feelings over the freckle are just that and it's not cancer. I hope I have overreacted like a crazy person. My arms were shaking from nerves. I didn't think my soul could take much more.

> —*Blog post, February 26, 2020*

We had a good chat. She looked at it and said, "I don't like it."

I told her to just take it all off. She looked at me, and I said, "I had a shitty year. Please don't tell me it's cancer."

She doesn't sugarcoat anything for me. She never has. She said she wanted me to see a dermatologist, and because of my cancer fatigue, she would put an urgent request in so I could just get it taken care of.

I asked her for the worst-case scenario. She looked right into my eyes and said, "If it is the worst stage melanoma, and the dermatologist cannot get enough skin around it for clear margins, you do chemotherapy. But I truly don't think this is that bad."

I said no. She called the dermatologist on her cell phone and asked her to call me back on my cell phone ASAP. Because my doctor is the best doctor. And she was looking out for me—including my mental state.

While she was typing notes into the computer, she asked how I was feeling after my year fighting DCIS. I told her about how I wished there were more support groups on the Eastside and that DCIS seems to be hiding everywhere. If you just open up, people come out of the woodwork who also have it. Or they know someone who did. I told her I was going to write a book about my journey.

She stopped me and said, "What makes you think you aren't qualified to start a support group on the Eastside?"

I answered that I thought a legitimate and safe support group needed an actual therapist (not just me waving my hands in the air), and maybe a nurse. She wrote down a number on a piece of paper and handed it to me. She said, "Here is your therapist to work with. Start a support group."

I stopped breathing. She got up, and I followed her out to see her receptionist (who I also missed in the year I hadn't seen her). She said, looking back at me, "You are destined to do great things, friend."

I could've cried. I didn't this time, but I could've. I chatted awhile with Ashley the receptionist and then got on my way. I stopped at the gym to do 1980s boot camp and then ran two miles to make the anger, fear, and worry tired.

> Should I cancel my Cancer-Free Boob Party? I was
> undecided. I do have a lot to celebrate. But I am still
> scared. And I am tired of being a downer for everyone
> around me. It's exhausting (to everyone) for sure. But I
> had to move forward. It just seems really stupidly unfair
> that DCIS didn't require chemotherapy, but a foot freckle
> would. I can't even handle that thought. Worst case
> scenario, I know. But after the year I had, it feels fair to
> think the worst and hope for the best.
>
> —*Blog post, February 26, 2020*

I did decide to celebrate with a party. My husband reserved a huge suite at a local hotel, and I invited nine friends to do a paint-and-sip with some appetizers, maybe go to dinner. We had prepared boob-themed party games, boob-related party prizes, and my friend Anna ordered boob cupcakes.

Melissa and her husband (who got quite excited about the whole process) made a boob bra-pong game, complete with boob ping-pong balls. They used all my old bras as targets to catch the balls. I also came up with boob bingo with breast markers. Prizes included a mug with boobs on it and several notebooks artistically decorated with boobs.

I was actually giddy when I woke up the morning of my party. I had to get the kids ready for their swim lessons, then go home to pack the supplies, and get a pretty party dress on! Hell, I figured I would even put makeup on for the first time in maybe three years. My kids helped me pick out jewelry, which is their favorite part about Mom going out for the night.

The day of my party was the first day of what eventually became a pandemic. On the news on the way to the party, we heard that one person had succumbed to COVID-19, the disease caused by a new virus discovered in China the same month I had my last surgery. So, there was already a bit of weariness in the eyes of my friends as they arrived, discussing what they heard about the beginning of the spread of the virus in our county. I would be lying if I said it didn't somehow dampen the early festivities. My husband required me to wipe down all the surfaces of the hotel room before guests arrived so we wouldn't get sick or spread the disease. That pretty much set the stage for the night. Too much champagne, a lot of painting, and a few boob games later, I was passed out in bed.

By the time of the party, friendships and dynamics had changed, matured, or fizzled out, but everyone showed up to celebrate the end of what had been a hard year. I wanted to thank everyone for the very different ways they helped me though my journey by preparing notes for each one of my party attendees. It was the least I could do.

The process of writing gratitude notes to each of my friends made me reflect on the people who could not be next to me through this journey but were also so helpful. My college friend Meg whose mother passed away from cancer years ago, was always an ear for me. I could feel her thinking of me across the miles. Kate and Lynn, both of whom I met while I was working as a historian in Massachusetts, were constantly on the other side of my phone, at all hours of the day and night.

At this point, I have let go of cancer, but I will not let go of the journey, because it taught me so much about myself, my strengths, and my weaknesses. I still think about that precipice in Alaska, and I carry with me the fear of looking down and the relief of standing at the bottom and looking up. I feel much the same way about DCIS. I cannot ever have breast cancer again. It's not physically possible. But I vividly remember all the emotions I carried with me on that journey, and the things I learned.

I learned how to let someone help and how to allow myself grace.

I learned how to choose my battles and how to talk to my children differently.

I learned how to manage expectations.

I am not willing to let go of the journey because I own it. The journey defines me. The cancer does not. There are days when I momentarily forget that I had cancer, and I know there will be longer moments in the future.

Did my ankle have cancer? No, turns out it was just an atypical mole. Crisis averted. Until the next one.

Though I finally threw that green plastic hospital bag that held my personal belongings away (five months after surgery), I still have those laughingly small ice packs from my first biopsy.

And I still have that stinky soap sitting on my shower shelf. I'm just not ready to throw it away yet.

EPILOGUE

I still have bad cancer days, even though I don't have cancer. I still have days where little things go incredibly wrong, and I collapse in a heap, wondering when life will get easier. I still have the dread that cancer is lurking around a corner, ready to jump on me when I least expect it. Though it has been suggested to me, I do not practice gratitude in every moment. I accept that my journey has been difficult but lucky. Difficult that I endured a cancer diagnosis and all the fear, anxiety and dread that accompany it; lucky that my treatment options did not include chemotherapy due to the stage cancer I had. But every day is a new day, and we move through it.

I went kayaking with Melissa one day and she said, "Did you name them yet?"

I laughed out loud and replied that I hadn't even thought about it.

She was asking me how I was. Not physically, but how I was as a whole person now that I am physically recovered. I have bad days, bad moments, but I recover and move forward.

> Then it happened. I relived the trauma. A friend I had become quite close within the first months of the pandemic got a call back about her very first mammogram. She turned 40 last week and one of the first things she did after blowing her candles out was make an appointment to have a mammogram. Since then, she was so full on anxiety that she could hardly function. She told me that at one point in the middle of the day, she saw an empty chair between her son and her husband and she flashed forward to a day when she wouldn't be there because she had died of cancer.
> "You think I am crazy."

"I don't at all. In fact, I had the same thoughts many times during my journey. It was when I took a picture of my kids and husband when we were on a hike. I broke down into tears immediately. To me, that was the picture of their lives without me."

All I wanted to do was to wrap my arms around her. But due to COVID, I cannot. I can't even get close. I wanted to tell her that everything was going to be OK. But I gave her statistics instead. And I told her that—though there is literally no reason she should have more of a risk of cancer—if she is diagnosed with cancer, it is curable.

I felt helpless. But I told her I would be here anytime of any day. And that I would never judge her for anything she was feeling.

And then it all hit me. Once I was out of the moment, it was all rushing back to me like March 2019, when I was waiting and making appointments and researching the cancer.org website and asking my friends who had been through multiple mammograms and callbacks. I was trying to step forward without sliding back.

So, I texted my friend throughout the next couple of days, distracting, checking in. And when she went in for her second mammogram, she found out that it was a cyst and it needed to be monitored every six months, but it wasn't anything to worry about. I congratulated her and told her I was relieved for her.

And that was true. But it was much more. I was sad and scared and tearful and relieved all at once, and I cried. I cried when I got the text that it was nothing to worry about.

I wish that had been my outcome. But it wasn't. And then I had to search my soul for something to be thankful for—didn't I?

—*Blog post, July 2, 2020*

Since my journey, and because I am so open about talking with people about boobs in general, I have learned from several women that you can request a mammogram appointment with a radiologist so they read your images while you sit there. If another scan needs to be taken, they take it then with no waiting in between. I cannot advocate for this more loudly. If I had known, I would have done this myself. And while I understand the challenging logistics of a radiologist being on call for all mammograms, I feel that lessening anxiety over waiting outweighs the logistical nightmare.

My breast cancer is gone but the journey will not ever be over. There are two bags of saline in my body that are a constant reminder I had cancer. There will be days in the future that I will forget for a while. Those stretches when I forget will become longer and longer with time. My takeaway from this Lump in the Road is that there is no one event that changes your life. It is a series of journeys and how you handle them that make you who you are.

It still surprises me how much, twenty-four years later, I remember about the precipice on which I stood in Alaska. It was an overcast day, but I could still see for miles. The mountain range in front of us was a beautiful, crisp, granite color with snowcapped tops. I can still feel how chilly I was and remember zipping up my fleece vest. I was scared to take a step and scared to make the wrong decision. But with support and determination, I moved forward. It was with those same feelings in my heart that I was able to approach and address my Lump in the Road with humility and practicality. Not everyone has the same diagnosis. Not everyone chooses the same path. Not everyone's journey is the same.

*   *   *

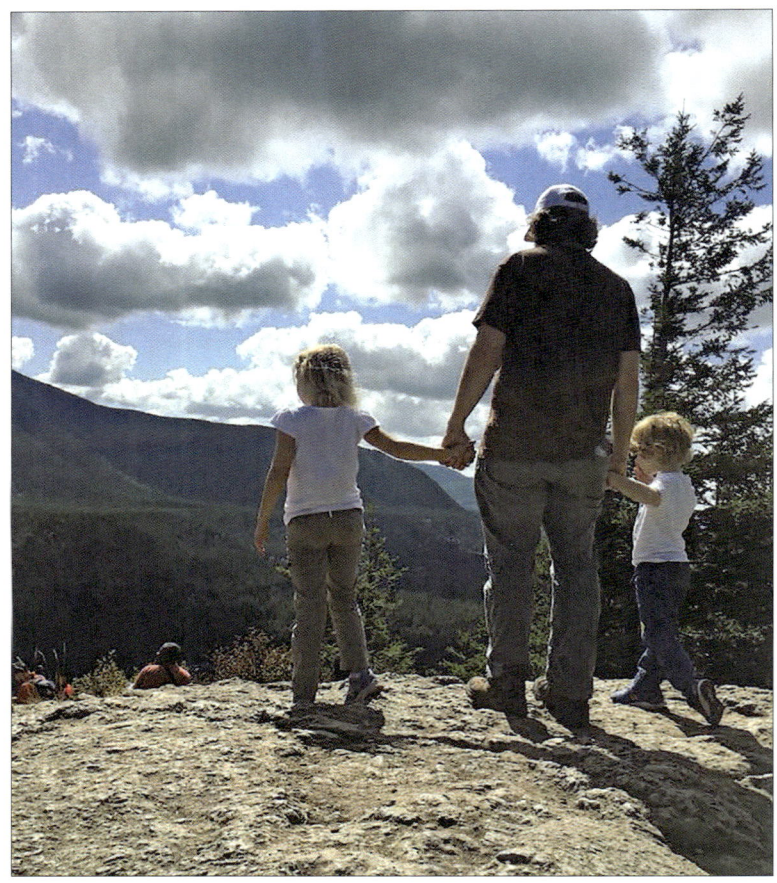

My family summited Rattlesnake Ledge, Washington, September 3, 2018. (This was before my cancer diagnosis, but we often found ourselves outside in nature.)

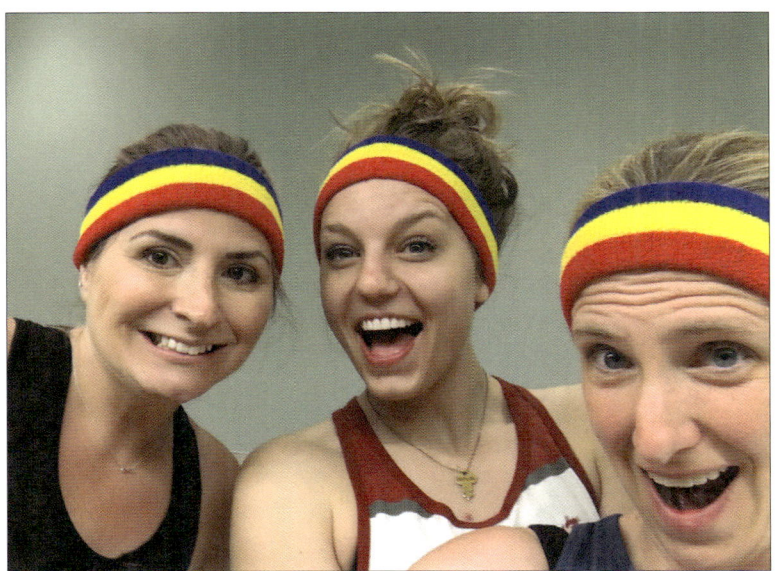

Bootcamp at the Sammamish YMCA with Andrea (left) and Ashley (middle), May 2019

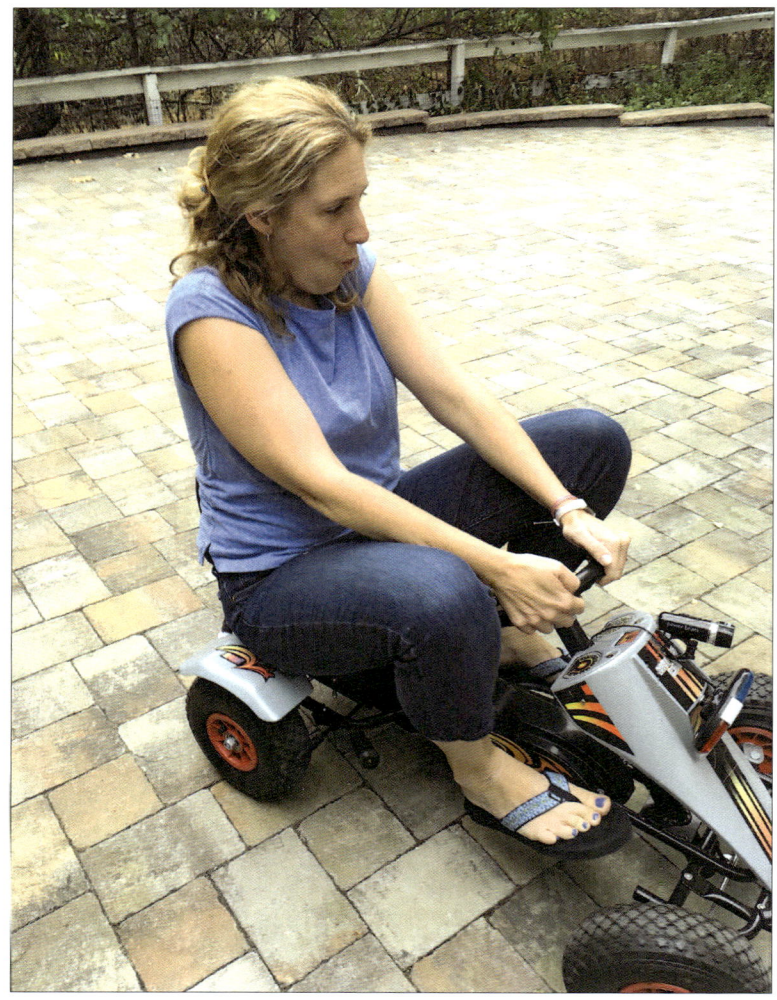

On a short trip to California, riding my kids' toys at my parents' house, October 2019

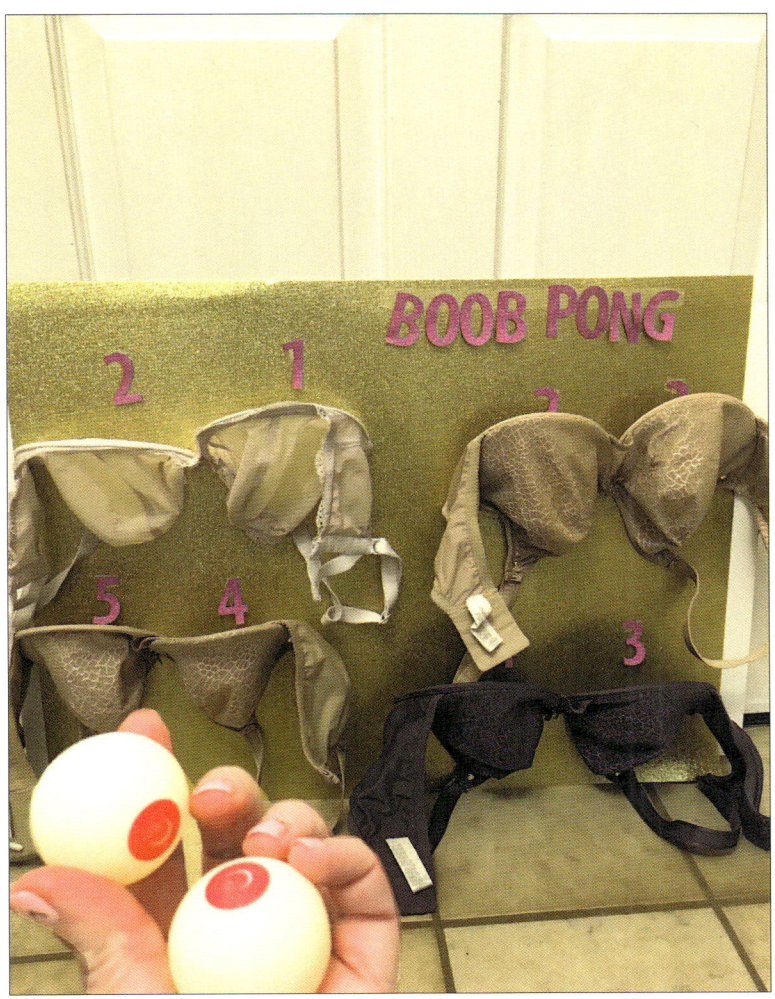

Boob Pong game for the Cancer-Free Party, February 29, 2020

ACKNOWLEDGMENTS

As I reflect on my tumultuous journey with DCIS, I realize that while I've gone through the ups and downs of diagnosis, treatment options, and recovery, I have just begun the road to recovery emotionally. And through it, I realize that my journey was one of the easier ones. I didn't have chemotherapy or radiation (or both). I have met many who have had those chemicals ravage their body to keep the cancer at bay, or even cure it. They are strong.

It hasn't even really sunk in that I am cancer-free. I have a long road ahead of me. And for that, I am thankful for the people I am surrounded with, near and far. I thank the friends who have supported me, filling my space with love, compassion, fear, positivity, anger, hope, confidence, and most importantly, humor. Without Sam, Andrea, Jessica, Ashley, Silvia, Eirlys, Julie, Meg, Brandy, Kelly, Lynn, and Melissa beside me, I would have been dragged down. Instead, I learned that when mostly negative energy flows around me, I can watch it dissipate, rather than get involved with it. You all got me through every day, every hour, every minute, and every second.

I saved a text message from a friend, and I looked at it almost daily for over a year. She wrote:

> We are writing this year off as soon as you're outta surgery....We turn a new decade with cancer-free boobs, and perky ones at that, and draw a line through cancer, my friend... *[emoji of middle finger]*

Anna, thank you for our friendship and the respect we have for one another. I love that we can disagree and still be friends. Discussions with you pushed me to make the right decision for me.

Kate P., thank you for asking so many questions and for encouraging me to find my voice in such a noisy world.

To my family practitioner, Dr. Jennifer Spence, thank you for always making my health a priority, for talking to me like a human, for treating me with respect, and speaking to me like a friend. Thank you for being the person who broke bad news to me in such a caring way.

A strong and meticulous thanks goes to the perfectionist attention and hands of Dr. Christine Lee, who led me through the options of a Stage 0 cancer diagnosis, calling me when I was worried about zings of pain, and answering my pages (and pages) of questions. You get extra points for being a real partner in my care and giving me the go-ahead to celebrate. The other half of my dynamic duo, Dr. Meghan Nadeau, was patient with my indecision and always had my personal best interest and preferences in mind. I gained such a huge respect for what you do every day and thank you for hearing me and respecting me. Your artistry will be appreciated for years to come. I am beyond lucky to have had two surgeons who treated me as a whole person.

To the doctor who performed my multiple biopsies, Dr. Kara Carlson, thank you for walking me through the procedure and laying out the worst-case scenarios. I appreciate your frankness.

Thanks to both Heidi Dishneau, ARNP, AOCNP, and Salima Hussain, RN, who answered many questions, spoke to me about holidays, welcomed me and calmed me throughout the multiple tests, surgeries, and procedures. And to Tifni Cloer, who shared her life with me as if we were friends, and who helped me with all that insurance paperwork. Knowing you all were on the other side of the phone or the office door always put me at ease.

To family and friends, near and far, who inquired about me, thought about me, offered to listen at any time, read drafts of my manuscript and offered love, thank you.

To my colleagues from NOLS Alaska 1996, you have unknowingly been with me in many ways through the years. Thank you for the assistance out of rivers, for a hand over the boulders, and for helping me find myself.

I thank my husband, who also did not ask for cancer, who stood by me, waited in uncomfortable waiting rooms, answered uncomfortable questions about what my boobs were doing and how they looked, emptied drains, and asked what I needed. I am sorry we had to do this, but I'm glad I didn't have to do this without you.

I am grateful for my parents, who listened to me vent every single day, and even though they were scared (but did not show it), knew that whatever the outcome at every step, I would get through it and come out on the other side of cancer.

To my mother-in-law, who graciously gave me her time and valuable opinions on several drafts of this memoir. Also, to Margaret and Colin Wood, who read an early draft and helped me attend a writer's workshop.

Thank you to Megan St. Marie and her staff at Modern Memoirs, Inc. for preserving my voice so it could be heard.

I am most thankful for two people, equally. My kids. If it hadn't been for them, that year would have been a year of more tears, more depression, and a spiral of despair I am not sure I would have been strong enough to come out of. They are the two people I focused on when I got scared. They were the ones for whom I want to model how to face and embrace fear, how to hope, and how to move on. I am grateful that they exist for me to be strong for.